INITIAL REPORT AND

PRELIMINARY RECOMMENDATIONS

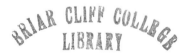

NATIONAL COMMISSION ON NURSING

An independent commission sponsored by
American Hospital Association, Hospital Research and Educational Trust,
and American Hospital Supply Corporation

840 North Lake Shore Drive, Chicago, Illinois 60611

ISBN 0-87914-058-5

Trust Catalog Number: 654100

25M-8/81-7709
10M-12/81-7881

Contents

Acknowledgment

This initial report has been written by the National Commission on Nursing. I wish to recognize the valuable contributions of all who provided the commission with data, information, and testimony; the commissioners and the organizations they represent; Gail Warden and Tita Corpuz, senior management consultants; Marjorie Beyers and Roberta Gutzwiller, commission staff; and Selby Toporek, of the American Hospital Association Division of Public Relations, who provided editorial assistance.

Representing a wide spectrum of issues, this report has been written to stimulate discussion and further deliberation about nursing-related issues. It is the commission's hope that it will not only create a dialog, but innovation and direction for the resolution of issues.

H. Robert Cathcart
Chairman
National Commission on Nursing

COMMISSIONERS
OF THE NATIONAL COMMISSION ON NURSING

CHAIRMAN

H. Robert Cathcart
President
Pennsylvania Hospital
Philadelphia, PA

COMMISSIONERS

Myrtle K. Aydelotte, R.N., Ph.D.
Executive Director
American Nurses' Association
Kansas City, MO

W. Daniel Barker
Administrator
Crawford W. Long Memorial
  Hospital of Emory
  University
Atlanta, GA

Sister Juliana Beuerlein, R.N.
Administrator
St. Joseph Hospital
Chicago, IL

Richard L. Bohy
Chairman
Assembly of Hospital Schools
  of Nursing
Chicago, IL
and
Vice-President
Sioux Valley Hospital
Sioux Falls, SD

Richard T. Chamberlin, M.D.
Medical Director
Bingham Associates Fund
Boston, MA

Georgeen H. DeChow, R.N.
Chairman of Nursing
Manatee Junior College
Bradenton, FL

JoAnna DeMeyer, R.N.
Assistant Administrator/
  Director of Nursing
St. Luke's Hospital
Boise, ID

Ruth S. Miller, R.N.
Standards Review Consultant
Lifemark Corporation
Houston, TX

Richard P. Moses
Representative
National Council of Hospital
  Governing Boards
Chicago, IL
and
Vice-Chairman of the Board
Tuomey Hospital
Sumter, SC

Marion I. Murphy, R.N., Ph.D.
Executive Director
American Association of
  Colleges of Nursing
Washington, DC

James H. Sammons, M.D.
Executive Vice-President
American Medical Association
Chicago, IL

W. Richard Scott, Ph.D.
Professor of Sociology
Stanford University
Stanford, CA

Margretta M. Styles, R.N., Ed.D.
Professor and Dean
University of California-
  San Francisco
School of Nursing
San Francisco, CA

Margaret E. Walsh, R.N.
Executive Director
National League for Nursing
New York, NY

SENIOR MANAGEMENT CONSULTANTS

Gail L. Warden
Chief Executive Officer
Group Health
  Cooperative of Puget Sound
Seattle, WA

Tita Corpuz, R.N.
Vice-President
American Hospital
  Association
Chicago, IL

COMMISSION STAFF

Marjorie Beyers, R.N., Ph.D.
Director
National Commission on
  Nursing
Chicago, IL

Roberta Gutzwiller, R.N.
Staff Specialist
National Commission on
  Nursing
Chicago, IL

Chapter

1

FRAMEWORK FOR RECOMMENDATIONS

THE COMMISSION'S CHARGE

The National Commission on Nursing, a forum of 30 commissioners, marks a unique multidisciplinary effort to address current nursing-related problems in the United States health care system. Commissioners represent a microcosm of the interdependent health care professionals and others who are concerned with health care and the relationships of nurses in the health care system. These 30 leaders in the field of nursing, hospital management, medicine, government, academia, and business, constitute a unique forum for the deliberation and consensus needed to resolve nursing problems as they relate to providing high quality patient care.

Charged with developing and implementing action plans for the future, the commission began its work in September, 1980. Its charge is as follows:

- Analyze the internal and external forces that influence the environment of nurses at work.
- Identify the effects of professional nursing issues on nursing practice in health care agencies.
- Assess the professional characteristics of nurses in relation to the organizational structure of health care agencies.
- Explore the motivation and incentives for nursing education and nursing practice.
- Analyze the relationship among education, nursing practice, and professional interaction in the health care agency.

1

- Develop a platform of issues to be dealt with in the commission activities.
- Plan methods to enhance the professional status and top management role of the nurse through:
  - research to define status and role
  - publication of information to describe or explain status and role in relation to health care
  - demonstration projects to provide models for problem resolution, development, and reshaping of relationships and structures in health care agencies

The overriding reason for the commission and its greatest concern as it continues its work is the nursing shortage. From the outset, it was recognized that the kinds of problems surrounding nursing would require a better understanding of the issues. This understanding necessitated opening up communications, involving the grass roots, and collecting data and information through public hearings, literature search, and review of state studies. The perceptions of the commissioners, those they come in contact with through their organizations, and others were also important to a better understanding of the issues.

The commission is an established mechanism for the exchange of information and ongoing communication among the commissioners, the organizations and constituencies they represent, and the grass roots level, and medicine, hospital administrators, and nursing. This mechanism had to be developed and supported before the work of the commission could begin.

In its efforts to explore the causes and effects of and potential solutions to current nursing-related issues and problems, in its first year of activity, the commission has established the forum necessary for consensus in decision-making. The leadership, diversity, and expertise represented by the commission provides a balanced perspective of nursing-related issues and problems in the context of society and of the health care system. In their several meetings, commissioners deliberated the problems and issues and examined data from a variety of sources. This *Initial Report* is the result of their deliberations to this point and presents their initial plan for action during the next two years of the commission's charter. Final recommendations will be published in 1983.

Data Collection

Following acceptance of its charge, the commission systematically began to examine and evaluate existing data sources. Relevant journal articles from 1975 to the present were reviewed and state studies and policy documents from 1977 to the present were located and examined. The valuable contributions of previous studies in nursing, the most recent being a study by the National Commission for the Study of Nursing and Nursing Education,* was apparent in both the review of journal articles and state studies. It was evident, however, that the rapidly-developing nursing issues and problems demanded current information and perspectives.

A series of public hearings were held, in an effort to look at the system in which nursing is practiced today. Many individuals, groups, and organizations responded to the commission's call for information through submission of documents, policy statements, data, and viewpoints. Nurses, physicians, health care administrators, researchers, politicians, representatives of professional health-related associations and organizations, consumers, and others provided testimony that supplied the commission with perspectives, data, and information on nursing-related issues as well as suggestions on how individuals, institutions, and organizations working together could confront and resolve current nursing-related problems within the health care system.

The public hearings, held in six major cities across the country, provided an opportunity for those concerned with nursing issues in each region of the country to testify. The commission also held two open forums with the AHA Center for Small or Rural Hospitals. Many of the persons submitting testimony offered views on how the commission could promote discussion and further study of nursing-related issues. They also offered suggestions for potential solutions. Following the hearings, the commission conducted an *Inventory of Innovative Programs and Projects* that were underway in health care institutions, academic institutions, and organizations.

Findings from sources of data, literature review, state studies, policy documents, the public hearings, and the *Inventory of Innovative Programs and Projects* were reviewed by the commissioners and formed the platform on which the commission's preliminary recommendations are based.

The highlights of these findings, the commission's preliminary recommendations, and future action plans are presented in this initial report. The preliminary recommendations reflect the areas in which a clear direction can be taken as well as those that require further study before final recommendations can be formed. The commission encourages responses to these recommendations. A final report will be published in 1983.

---

*Lysaught, J.P., director. *An Abstract For Action*. New York: McGraw-Hill, 1970. The National Commission for the Study of Nursing and Nursing Education was supported by the W.K. Kellogg Foundation, Avalon Foundation, and a private individual from 1967-1970.

Forming the Recommendations

Nursing is an integral part of the dynamic and complex health care system in this country. In developing preliminary recommendations, the commissioners focused on those that will strengthen nursing's ability to respond to the challenges posed by the changing health care system.

The commissioners found the present situation of nursing to be complex, involving numerous groups and organizations. Bringing various organizations and their leaders into a single forum has brought these issues to a common ground and has established a shared level of knowledge about the issues. The increasing interdependence of health care professionals within the health care system requires this common level of knowledge about issues and problems, if they are to be resolved.

In addition to the interdependence of health care professionals, the commission has been conscious of the fact that nursing takes place in a variety of practice settings. Acute care, rehabilitation, long term care, community and public health, school health, and industry are examples. The movement toward multinstitutional arrangements for health care and the broadened base of nursing practice in the health care system also were recognized.

The hospital, however, has been the dominant health care corporation in the total system and the largest percentage of nurses is in hospitals. The intensive level of care, the acute nature of patient needs, and the fact that two-thirds of all practicing nurses are in hospitals were factors pointed out in testimony at the public hearings. In this light, it was decided to focus primary attention on hospital nursing. Despite the fact that the preliminary recommendations of the commission focus on the elements needed to strengthen hospital nursing, many of the conclusions can be applied to other settings in which nurses practice.

In addition to differences in practice settings, there are regional differences in nursing practice in the United States. When viewed from the national perspective, the issues are more similar than different. In this preliminary report, the commission has outlined a direction for change targeted to the national perspective. There are important steps to be taken to strengthen nursing that should simultaneously strengthen the entire health care system.

The Major Issues

The National Commission on Nursing, in addressing nursing issues and problems, focused on the system in which nursing is practiced today rather than on defining nursing practice. It was agreed that the definition of nursing practice is the responsibility of the profession. A large body of data and information yielded multiple factors

4

related to the current shortage of nurses. The factors presented in testimony were typical of those presented in other data sources. More than 40 different factors frequently and consistently were mentioned in testimony. Salaries, flexible scheduling, nurse- physician relationships, the image and status of nurses and their roles in decision-making, career mobility, nursing education, and the relationship of nursing education and nursing practice were foremost in the long list.

All of these factors were abstracted from testimony and summarized into five major categories of issues that also represent those found in the commission's literature review. They are:

- Status and image of nursing, including changes in the nursing role in response to new variations in health care delivery and professional growth as well as the corresponding changes in interprofessional relationships and public image
- Interface of nursing education and practice, including current and potential models for basic and graduate education and continuing nursing education to prepare nurses for practice and professional interaction in health care delivery
- Effective management of the nursing resource, including the mix of organizational factors required for nursing job satisfaction (such as the issues of staffing, scheduling, salary and benefits, support services, modes of care delivery, and career development) as well as manpower planning and recruitment and retention strategies
- Relationships among nursing, medical staff, and hospital administration, including nurses' ability to participate through organizational structures in decision-making as it relates to nursing care, the value and development of collegial relationships among health care professionals, and the development and operation of interdisciplinary patient care teams
- Maturing of nursing as a self-determining profession, including nursing's right and responsibility to define and determine the nature and scope of its practice, the need for and role of nursing leadership, the potential of collective action to increase decision-making in nursing practice, and the need for unity in the nursing profession

KEY RELATIONSHIPS

As indicated by the five major categories of issues raised at the public hearings, the current problems and issues in nursing are complex. In an effort to develop a framework that synthesized the issues, without losing sight of the important critical factors, the commission first identified a number of key relationships that link nurses with one another and with other groups.

These relationships were noted to cluster in three broad areas; nursing practice, nursing education, and nursing and the public. Although separated for discussion and analysis, these areas are interdependent. Indeed, the interdependence of all of nurses' relations in practice, education, and in dealing with the public is a key element in the complexity of the issues and problems affecting nursing.

Within each of these three broad areas, the cluster of key relationships includes:

Nursing Practice: relations between nurses and

- physicians
- health care administrators
- health care institutions
- the nursing profession
- unions
- supplementary staffing agencies

Nursing Education: relations between

- the nursing profession and education
- nursing education and nursing practice

Nursing and the Public: relations between nurses and

- state governments
- federal government

These key relationships were identified by the commission as most helpful to understanding the desired outcomes of the commission's work, as embodied in the commission's charge. These desired outcomes are:

- retention of nurses in practice
- job satisfaction
- maintaining and increasing the competence of nurses in practice
- maintaining and improving the quality of nursing care

By dealing with the basic issues in nursing education, practice, and public policy initiatives directed toward nursing, some of the more specific proposed solutions, such as flexible scheduling, mix of staff, and career ladders, come into a broader focus. It is the commissioners' belief that useful and practical solutions to nursing-related problems are addressed best from the long-term view and from analysis of the underlying relations and structures. Nursing now is at a critical point in its history. Nursing's future development and that of the health care system in which nursing practice takes place will be determined by directions chosen and by actions taken now.

Chapter

2

NURSING PRACTICE

Nurses, health care administrators, physicians, trustees, and others have different perceptions of nursing roles and functions. Nursing care is an essential service that nurses provide in a variety of settings. Although they are accountable for nursing care, nurses at all levels often have insufficient decision-making authority in management of patient care and in other areas of the environment in which nurses practice. Some nurses are seeking extra-institutional mechanisms to gain control over their practice, there is lack of agreement about nursing roles and functions. There is no cohesive professional body that speaks for and is accepted by all nurses.

Key relationships in the area of nursing practice are between:

- Nurses and physicians and nurses and health care administrators
- Nurses and health care institutions
- Nurses and the nursing profession
- Nurses and unions, and nurses and supplementary agencies

NURSES AND PHYSICIANS;
NURSES AND HEALTH CARE ADMINISTRATORS

The Environment
Nurses, physicians, and health care administrators share the concern for high quality patient care. National attention has been drawn to nursing because of the effects of widespread shortages of nurses. Recent state studies[1] show that vacancies in budgeted registered nurse positions range from eight to 17 percent in

hospitals alone. Long term care facilities and community health agencies, and schools of nursing also report shortages of qualified registered nurses for clinical, teaching, and management roles. The average national turnover rate for registered nurses in hospitals is 30 percent.[2] This high turnover rate further constrains health care agencies' ability to provide high quality patient care.

Many health care agencies, especially hospitals, have used expedient and often costly interventions to recruit and retain nurses. Bonuses for recruiting staff, full pay for shortened work hours, cash and benefit incentives, and bonuses for remaining in employment were reported in both the National Commission on Nursing's Public Hearings and in the review of nursing-related literature. Shortages prevail despite these interventions. Testimony at the public hearings and the literature review indicate that many short-term measures did not touch on the fundamental unresolved nursing issues. One of the most fundamental of these is lack of recognition for nurses' worth in patient care.

Perceptions of Nurses' Roles
Both testimony and review of the literature indicate that physicians and health care administrators often do not fully understand the role of nurses in patient care. Traditional and outdated images of nurses are thought by many authors to impede acceptance of these current roles.[3-7] Victorian stereotypes of nurses, traditional male-female relationships, and traditional organizational delivery systems for nursing care were cited as barriers that must be overcome if nurses are to be recognized for their practice. Some physicians and health care administrators perceive nurses to be over-educated for their roles and do not support increasing nurses' decision-making in nursing practice.[8-9] Others believe, however, that there are insufficient numbers of nurses with adequate preparation to meet the demand for acute care. Increased need for nursing care, as reported in testimony and in recent literature, stems from new types of family units, increasing numbers of elderly persons, changing disease patterns, expansion of technology and information, and the growth of specialization in health care. Patients' increased knowledge about health care and the broadened scope of health care benefits in many employee reimbursement programs are two other frequently mentioned factors that have increased demand for nursing care. Physicians testifying in the commission's public hearings considered clinical competence of nurses to be essential to quality patient care, and a necessary aspect of establishing complementary nurse-physician roles in patient care, based on mutual trust and respect.

The need for clinical competence of nurses to be recognized

and more fully utilized in patient care also was clearly expressed in the literature.[10-15] In reporting findings of their extensive study of the image of nurses, Kalisch and Kalisch noted that efforts to improve the image of nurses should be related to improved health care services.[16] Stereotypes that nurses and physicians have of each other's roles were shown to be related to experience and socialization in a study conducted in two Seattle hospitals.[17] There is strong indication from both testimony and literature review that changing societal needs for care and changing health care technology increasingly require sharing the knowledge and authority by health care professionals.

Nurse-Physician Collaborative Practice
Shared responsibility for patient care between nurses and physicians also was the focus of the National Joint Practice Commission (NJPC) established in 1971 to examine the roles and functions of nurses and physicians, and to work to remove sources of professional differences affecting their collaboration.[18]

The NJPC definition of collaborative practice is based on elements of the nurse-physician relationship including care of the same group of patients, a joint practice committee, formal and informal communications, joint determination of nonclinical actions relevant to patient care by nurses, physicians, and hospital administration; acceptance of individual clinical judgments; joint evaluation of patient care according to jointly established standards, continuing education, administrative support, and patient satisfaction.[19]

Efforts of the NJPC to improve nurse-physician relationships were directed to hospitals because ... "there the majority of nurses gain their clinical experience and continue their careers, and there the greatest number of nurses and physicians are associated with each other in providing patient care. Significant changes in their relationship will affect more nurses and physicians than changes in any other setting, and will in time be reflected in nurse-physician relationships everywhere."[20]

The NJPC conducted demonstration projects in four prototype United States hospitals to examine the effectiveness of attempts to develop collaborative practice in hospitals. Evaluation of these projects suggests that collaborative practice efforts result in improved quality of patient care and in satisfaction of both nurses and physicians with their practice. Features of effective collaborative practice established as a result of the NJPC's demonstration projects include a collaborative practice committee with equal representation by nurses and physicians, with administration's support. In this committee, individual clinical nursing decisions are made using medical and nursing consultations.

The commission's *Inventory of Innovative Programs and Projects* contains descriptions of these nurse-physician collaborative practice committees that resulted in increased independent clinical decision-making by nurses and definition of nurses' and physicians' complementary roles in patient care to improve the quality of patient care. Also described is a visiting program for first year medical students to educate physicians about nursing roles and to establish positive attitudes about the complementary roles of nurses and physicians.[21] Interdisciplinary committees and conferences for nurses and physicians were described by a number of authors as effective in improving patient care.

Interdisciplinary Health Care Teams
Recent literature also contains information about emerging interdisciplinary health care teams. One example is care of oncology patients by a team of nurses, hematologists, and oncology medical specialists;[24] another is care of critically ill persons by a team of surgeons, critical care nurses, a cardiac nurse coordinator, psychiatric social worker, medical sociologist, pulmonary function therapist, physician therapist, and dietitian.[25] Interdisciplinary teams reported as successful in these examples.

Problems emerging in the development of interdisciplinary health care teams also have been described. Some physicians do not agree with the view that the practice of medicine is a team activity.[26] The quest for leadership among team members, lack of procedure and processes by which teams carry out their activities, energy spent dealing with interdisciplinary team members' personal conflicts rather than on patient care[27-30] and lack of support during the change to interdisciplinary teams for conflict resolution,[31-33] are problems described.

Although patterns of professional interaction are changing, nurses and physicians consistently are included in all of the interdisciplinary health care teams described. The relationships between these two groups may well determine their relationships with other health care professionals.

Health Care Administrators' Key Roles
The key role of health care administrators in administrative support of collaborative practice and interdisciplinary health care also was emphasized in testimony at the public hearings. It was said that development of a collaborative approach to patient care should have its beginnings in basic educational preparation and socialization of physicians, nurses, and health care administrators into their professional roles. It was stated that increased patient acuity requires improved communication and cooperation among nurses,

physicians, and health care administrators with each professional group attending to different aspects of care.

Nurse Administrators' Key Roles

The nurse administrator's position and influence in the institution were factors reported by staff nurses to be important to their job satisfaction and feeling of recognition. The ability of the nurse administrator to succeed in shaping staff nurses' participation in patient care was viewed as directly dependent on the nurse administrator's ability to work cooperatively on a professional basis with the hospital administrative and medical staff. The testimony that nurse administrators who participate in policy-making bodies in the institution are in a better position to influence nurse satisfaction was supported in the literature. The importance of the organizational setting in influencing the relationship between nurses and physicians has been demonstrated in a study conducted by Alberts.[34]

Organization of Nursing Care Delivery

Need to change organizational modes for nursing care delivery also was emphasized in both testimony and the literature review. Until care in hospitals is reorganized and nurses become more assertive and committed to their goals, professional nursing practice will not be recognized.[35] Professionalism in nursing is hindered by "allegiance to hospital rules rather than to professional principles."[36] Revamping attitudes, enlightening colleagues, and administrative and medical staff recognition of nurses as professionals are needed to capture nursing's expertise in patient care.[37-41] These examples from the literature were echoed in testimony as reasons for nurse-physician-health care administrator's shared participation in top management of health care institutions.

Nursing's Involvement in Policy-Making

Further evidence of the importance of nursing's involvement in policy-making at the institutional level was given in testimony. Presenters indicated that outdated management methods and traditional organizational modes of nursing care delivery were barriers to nurses' abiility to use their expertise in patient care effectively. They desire self-governance and self-discipline in their practice but do not see that they can gain decision-making authority and accountability for their practice unless they are represented by a competent nurse administrator in executive management, the level of management reporting directly to the chief executive officer. It was assessed in testimony that the cost of failure to change the institution's philosophy about and recognition of nursing practice was great. Decreased quality of patient care, high turnover rates of nurses, and dollar costs to the institution for recruitment, orientation, and bed closures were cited.

Factors in Nurse Satisfaction

Intellectual stimulation and a sense of achievement were found to be important factors in nurse satisfaction in a study in which more than 40 percent of 1,000 nurses surveyed had dropped out of nursing.[42] Half of these nurses dropped out after five years of initial employment. Many moved about from job to job with no promotion because of lack of ability to change their conditions of practice. Other researchers found that variety in functions, good communication among professionals in patient care matters, promotional opportunity, and participation in decision making resulted in nurse satisfaction.[43] In another study, autonomy in work and recognition in salary and personal achievement were found to be important factors in nurse retention.[44]

The high cost of turnover also was reported. One researcher found that a 61 percent turnover in new graduate nurses cost an estimated 20 million plus loss of efficiency, decreased quality patient care, and immeasurable personal cost to nurses.[45] In this study, recognition was the most frequently mentioned satisfier for nurses; achievement and successful completion of tasks, also were mentioned frequently. A nurse administrator attributes an 11-percent decrease in staff nurse turnover to managerial and organizational changes[46] allowing participatory management and committee structures for nurse decision-making at all levels of the organization.

Organizational Change

Examples of organizational changes underway were reported in the commission's *Inventory of Innovative Programs and Projects*. One effort is a statewide educational program that deals with creating a new hospital environment and that requires attendance by the triad of nurse administrator, health care administrator, and a physician leader. Another is formation of a nursing executive committee which parallels the Medical Executive Committee of many institutions. Membership on the committee includes nurse administrators, staff nurses, health care administrators, and trustees. Standing subcommittees of this committee promote a collaborative approach to health care, and provide for while allowing nursing to control establishment of nursing care standards by nurses.

Analysis

Despite the fact that nursing historically has accepted a broad re-

14

sponsibility for patient care, for the first time, nurses are saying they lack the necessary authority and involvement to carry out their professional responsibilities. Nurses are involved in and perform a major role in the implementation of the total plan of care; they participate in the formulation and integration of the medical plan of care. Nursing participation in both clinical and managerial decisions is necessary to ensure the delivery of high quality health care and to provide a more satisfying environment for professionals. Supportive interprofessional relationships among nurses, health care administrators, and physicians are crucial in nursing's participation in clinical and managerial decisions. Physicians and health care administrators must recognize that their relationship with the nursing profession in any given practice setting may well set the tone for their relationships with other health care professionals.

Recommendations

1. Nurses and physicians participate in a collaborative partnership in the provision of patient care. To assure excellent patient care, nurses should be included in the clinical decision-making process and must have sufficient authority and must accept responsibility for their professional practice.
2. Physicians must accept the responsibility to promote the recognition of the knowledge and abilities of nurses to make decisions in patient care.
2. Health care administrators in all practice settings have an obligation to establish a suitable environment for nurses to practice their profession. Establishing the environment must include involvement of the nurse administrator as part of the top management team, assuring that nursing participates in policy development and in management decisions at every level of the organization.
4. Trustees, health care administrators, and physicians must ensure that nurses are accorded the professional recognition to provide clinical nursing services to patients.

NURSES AND HEALTH CARE INSTITUTIONS

The Administrators' View
Health care administrators in individual hospitals and in multi-institutional settings keenly are aware of the importance of a stable

15

nursing staff for providing quality patient care. Testimony in the public hearings substantiated the connection between high quality patient care and a stable nursing staff. High rates of nurse turnover, bed closures owing to shortages of nurses, and other effects of the current nursing situation are all felt by health care administrators. Increased cost of nurse recruitment, high costs of orientation, and costs of incentives to enhance nurse retention in an environment of cost containment in health care were reported to be a major problem for health care administrators. Many of these administrators, in sincere attempts to comprehend the nursing issues, have been confounded by failure of short-term solutions to rectify the current nursing situation.

The Nurses' View
Nurses, on the other hand, indicated at the public hearings that the most tangible evidence of lack of recognition of their worth in patient care is found in low and compressed salaries that nurses receive. Despite great variance in their levels of educational preparation and experience, all nurses are paid at about the same salary. Registered nurses earn only a few dollars more per hour than licensed practical nurses or nurse aides. It was shown in one study that only about 12 percent of hospitals pay nurses who have baccalaureate degrees more than registered nurses who have lesser education.[47] Testimony at the public hearings, literature review and state studies indicate that nurses who have 10 to 20 years' experience earn about the same salary as newly graduated registered nurses. Nurses promoted to management positions may earn less than do staff nurses or head nurses. The majority of nurses who testified at the public hearings thought that their salaries were inadequate for the amount of responsibility they accepted in patient care.

Less tangible, but equally important to nurses, is their ability to make decisions in patient care and in mattters affecting their practice. Those presenting testimony emphasized that the quality of practice and rewards in the practice setting must be increased to retain nurse employees. The strong sense of nurses that they neither can practice nursing effectively nor make decisions about matters affecting their practice was expressed by many as lack of professional autonomy. Participation in decision-making, professional recognition, and the opportunity for career advancement also were found to be important satisfiers for nurses in several studies.[48-52]

The Practice Setting
Wide variations in institutional practice settings for nurses were described in testimony about nurses' employment. At one end was a

description of a newly designed organizational structure that promotes the independent practice of nursing—professionally educated and credentialed nurses will apply for nursing practice privileges, be in control of and accountable for their practice, be reimbursed on the basis of quality and quantity of care given, and be self-governing and self-disciplining. At the other end was the testimony of a hospital administrator who described inadequacies of middle management in many hospitals that lead to lack of standards for support systems to which nursing is particularly vulnerable. Nurses, "because of the primacy of their accountability," assume responsibility for performing these support services. Consequently, patients are deprived of the professional nursing care that only nurses are educated to perform, because inordinate time is spent performing essential but non-nursing functions. The strong call for nursing's governance of its clinical practice presented in testimony is related to and consistent with the equally strong call for freeing nurses from nonnursing tasks.

Organization of Nursing

A wide range of approaches was reported in testimony concerning the institutional organization of nursing services. Many nurse administrators reported that their titles and positions place them at the level of executive management. Others indicated that the nursing department was subordinated to an administrative structure that failed to accord nurses the authority for nursing functions or participation in institutional decisions affecting nursing care.

Participative Management

Emerging forms of participative management for nurses were described. The philosophy of participative management for a multihospital system employing 4,000 to 5,000 nurses was presented in testimony. Elements in this philosophy were a spirit of collaboration, consensus-seeking, and cooperation based on respect for each others' worth; vesting decision-making authority so that persons retain as much influence as possible over their work and working environment; and accountability for how the authority was exercised in fulfilling goals and objectives for patient care.

Some nurse administrators testified that there are discrepancies between their executive titles and their actual involvement in executive management. There was general agreement among them that nursings' involvement in decision-making should include participation in administrative committees; budget preparation, policy development, and other management activities. Some believed that nursing should have access to the board of trustees.

Educational Preparation for Nurse Managers

To participate effectively in executive management, it generally was agreed that master's level preparation is essential. The nurse manager's role was presented in testimony as a complex and demanding role that requires strong leadership skills, fiscal management, creativity, and an understanding of nursing care and business administration. The shortage of nurse managers prepared by education to manage the increasing responsibilities of the management unit, was presented as a major problem in both testimony and in the literature. In 1977, only 27 percent of nurse administrators in the United States held a master's degree. The baccalaureate degree was the highest level of educational preparation for 24 percent. [53]

Promotions to administrative positions as reported in testimony, were most often based on clinical skills or seniority. Although those presenting testimony supported new organizational designs that could result in important changes in the practice of nursing and substantial increases in the contribution of nurses in hospitals, they emphasized the need to prepare nurse managers for the responsibilities of providing quality patient care, evaluating that care, and establishing an environment in which nurses could make maximum use of their skills. Classifying patients according to acuity of need, adapting staffing to these needs, balancing costs, meeting ever-changing regulatory standards, and maintaining high quality patient care in cooperation with other health professionals, require adequate educational preparation. The imperative that nursing professionals and hospital administrators together address the problem of preparing nurse managers for their roles was emphasized in testimony.

Organizational Structure for Nursing

Testimony emphasized the advantages associated with establishing the nursing department as a distinct management unit for clinical nursing practice within the institution. In this unit, nurses would function as professionals with full authority over their practice. Examples of self-governance in such a management unit were given in testimony and found in the literature. Self-governance is defined within the nursing profession as their ability to establish a distinct management entity with a high level of self-determination over the standards of practice and autonomy within the practice setting. Professional nurses desire to exercise their decision-making capability to manage nursing care according to shifting patient and institutional requirements. Established organizational structures that govern nursing as simply another hospital department are not adequate for the rapidly changing and complex patient care environment.

Development of self-governance in a management unit for nursing, reported in both testimony and in the literature, involves structuring nursing's participation in management. In many institutions, nursing bylaws are being developed to promote nurses' participation. Some have nursing bylaws circumscribed to the nursing department.[54-55] Others report a nursing staff organization governed by bylaws that are separate from nursing management and provide for direct accountability to the board of trustees.[56-58] Staff and practice privileges, confirmation of education and certification, review of clinical work, remedies for substandard practice, quality assurance mechanisms, requirements for continuing education, participation in educational preparation of nursing students, and involvement in research to improve patient care are features of many bylaws structures.[59]

Other forms of nursing participation reported were establishment of a nursing assembly or nursing management council for decision-making in patient care.[60-62] Committee structures that provide for staff nurse participation in decisions that affect their practice and employment were described in the *Inventory of Innovative Programs and Projects*. Several authors relate new forms of organizational structures for nursing to shifting organizational relationships. The nurse managers' authority for institutional level decision-making, staff nurses' authority for patient care decisions, and relationships with physicians and health care administrators are changing toward a new organizational equilibrium in their view.[62-68] It was stressed in testimony, as well as in the literature review, that deliberation and consensus about new organizational structures requires combined collaborative efforts of nurses, health care administrators, physicians, and trustees.

Organization of Nursing Care Delivery
The staff nurse role was presented in testimony as being dependent not only on the numbers and types of nurses, but on support services for housekeeping, information systems, and other departments that support patient care. Organizational modes for nursing care delivery were viewed as defining staff nurse functions. Variants of these modes were reported to exist according to the time period in a 24-hour cycle, day of the week, available staff, and patient acuity in a given institution. The most frequently used modes, functional, team, and primary nursing care were reported rarely to exist in the pure, text definitions. Staff nurses cited that in any organization, they feel more supported in their nursing care roles and in relations with other health care professionals when the nurse administrator effectively represented nursing in the institution.

Primary Nursing Care

Primary Nursing Care was the organizational mode of nursing care delivery nurses perceived to be most satisfying, according to testimony at the public hearings. In this mode, staff nurses accept responsibility for and are accountable for individualized patient care for a group of patients. Considered to enhance the professionalism of nursing and to improve the quality of patient care, primary nursing also was presented as cost-effective.

Although there was strong support for primary nursing care as a desirable organizational mode, an opposing view was presented in testimony. Primary nursing care, in this view, was described as contradictory to the management principles that duties and responsibilities should be delegated to the lowest level of personnel competent to fulfill them. This argument reflects the labor force view of nursing. Staff nurses, however, considered this emphasis on staffing and task orientation, rather than on quality nursing care, as stress producing. "Nurses are expected to have infinite elasticity, caring for more patients than is reasonable or safe. Requests for increased staffing are countered by the statement that the nurse is costly and non-income producing."[69] Economic constraints attributed to third-party reimbursement inadequacies in both acute care hospitals and in nursing homes were reported by staff nurses as contradictory to the purposes of these institutions to provide high quality patient care for which nurses have 24-hour-a-day accountability.

Evaluation of the effectiveness of primary nursing care was reported in the literature. Improved satisfaction for patients, nurses, and physicians were reported.[70-75] Earlier patient discharge, improved quality of patient care, and similar or lower costs, were among other positive results reported. One can infer that there is a direct relationship between continuity of care and satisfaction of nurses. Other organizational modes for nursing care delivery may accomplish these results if they eliminate other factors, such as floating from one area to another, which nurses believe interferes with continuity of care. Hospitals introducing primary nursing care have reported increasing numbers of registered nurse staff; some studies show that costs in those institutions appear to be the same or lower when compared with other modes of nursing care delivery because of better utilization of nursing competencies.[76-80]

It is important to note that the majority of evaluations of the outcomes of primary nursing care are descriptive; few studies have been completed in more than a single hospital. Results are somewhat conflicting. One author refers to high start-up costs for planned educational programs for nurses, physicians, and health care administrators to assist them in developing new roles, evaluation methods, and support systems necessary for primary nursing care.[81] No conclusive differences were found in job satisfaction for nurses in primary nursing care as compared with those of nurses in team nursing by one researcher; another found that nurses on primary nursing care units had lower absentee and resignation rates than those on nonprimary units, but that job satisfaction measures used in the study did not vary between the two groups.[82]

New Organizational Modes

Despite the conflicting evidence about primary nursing care, nurses presenting testimony agreed that structures for organization of nursing care delivery should allow for more personalized patient care and professional decision-making opportunities for nurses. It also was agreed that these should be cost-effective, promote the professional stature of nursing, and meet outcome criteria of improved patient care and nurse satisfaction. In one institution, nurses developed their own modes of nursing care delivery according to parameters defined by an oversight committee. These nurses reported optimal patient care, employee satisfaction, and patient satisfaction with care received when nurses on each patient care area selected their own mode of care delivery.

Failure of institutions to establish organizational modes that promote professional nursing practice was reported in testimony to be related to staffing and scheduling problems that are of immediate concern to nurses. Overwork, long hours, working different shifts in a given week, and floating from one unit to another were thought by staff nurses, to lead to increased resignations. Increased recognition of nurses' professional role in care and creativity in designing organizational modes for nursing care that focused on the quality of patient care rather than on numbers of staff allotted in the budget for each patient care unit could, in these nurses' view, break the cycle of inadequate staffing and scheduling problems.

Nurses also reported that structures for patient care delivery should include innovations in systems designed to decrease time nurses spend in nonnursing tasks. Programs to provide support services for nurses, such as monitoring technicians and nurse extenders, and programs in which unit managers, working under nursing management, perform nonnursing activities were reported in the commission's *Inventory of Innovative Programs and Projects.*

A few comprehensive projects were reported in which the entire management unit for nursing was restructured. In these projects, the organizational mode of nursing care delivery was related to support services for patient care, the environment of care including staff nurses' opportunity for decision-making, and a system for career advancement. Mechanisms to define and develop the relationships of nurses as professionals in the organization were targeted as essential in these projects.

Career Advancement

As nurses' professionalism increasingly is being recognized, the lack of opportunity for career advancement is apparent. It was acknowledged in testimony that 40-50 percent of the hospital's total personnel budget is designated for nursing, that nurses are the basic component in the delivery of increasingly complex care, and that budget, personnel policies, salaries, and benefits, must be viewed in a composite. Opportunities for professional growth in the institutional setting were reported to rank high on the list of factors important in nurse satisfaction. It also was reported that designing these opportunities requires involvement of fiscal, nursing, personnel, and administrative departments.

Several existing and developing patterns of career ladders were described in testimony. Two examples were levels of practice based on distinct levels of clinical practice, from beginning practitioner skills to advanced skills, and a clinical progression program based on organized peer review for merit advancement. In these programs, clinical competency was recognized and salaries were increased, based on evidence of competence and contribution to patient care. Increased salary based on documented clinical competence provides an answer to the severe wage compression nurses experience.

Common features of levels of practice or clinical advancement systems reported in the literature include the need to define competencies commensurate with standards of nursing practice, develop personnel policies for promotion, and place staff into appropriate levels once they are defined.[83-87] Evaluation programs, educational programs, and peer review mechanisms were other common features. In the reports of career advancement programs in employment settings, there was variation in educational qualifications recognized in promotion systems and in the extent of educational programs provided to help nurses achieve greater competency.

Several authors reported the effects of career advancement programs. One author indicated that cost-savings may result from improving qualifications of nurses and from relating levels of competence to nursing care functions. Increased decision-making authority, job satisfaction, and professionalism were reported.[88] Elimination of the traditional supervisor role was anticipated by one author.[89] Career advancement programs, such as levels of practice, have not been in existence long enough to evaluate the long-term results. It is apparent, however, from testimony and from literature review that comprehensive planning for career advancement programs includes elements of education, personnel policies for promotion, budgetary considerations and, most importantly, the organizational mode for nursing care delivery.

Analysis

Effective use of registered nurses, to realize their potential for nursing care, will benefit the entire health care system. Many traditional organizational structures in health care agencies do not accommodate nurses as professionals. Staff nurses, although accountable for direct patient care, often are managed like conventional workers under nonprofessional working conditions and are expected to perform organizationally-defined tasks that often include nonnursing functions, such as housekeeping. Differences in educational preparation and specialized competency of nurses are not recognized within health care settings. Salaries are not commensurate with responsibilities of nurses as professionals and reflect severe wage compression. Institutions do not provide for career advancement in nursing practice.

Changes in organizational structures are essential. Restructuring the organization of nursing care in health care agencies will result in improved patient care and improved job satisfaction. The provision of appropriate support services will promote effective use of nursing in patient care. Organizational recognition of career advancement sequences, with equitable benefits, will result in increased retention of nurses in the profession.

Recommendations

1. Nursing should be structured as a clinical and management entity that promotes professional nursing practice, and the nurse manager should be responsible for assuring that adequate resources are provided to maintain quality nursing care.
2. The management unit should be led by a nurse administrator who is qualified by education and experience to promote, develop, and maintain an organizational climate conducive to professional nursing practice and effective management of the nursing resource.
3. Salaries, benefits, and educational opportunities for nurses should be developed to ensure that they are commensurate with responsibilities of nurses as professionals.
4. The quality of supporting services to the patient care unit is a major determinant in the effectiveness of the delivery system and the satisfaction of the professionals working in the system. In order to ensure a high level of quality support services, nursing, as part of the management team, actively should participate in the establishment of a standard of quality of support services.

NURSES AND THE NURSING PROFESSION

Nursing's Professional Image
A professional image for nursing will be determined by its ability to meet the standard criteria for a profession, and the public trust that goes with professionalism. Public trust will be promoted by establishing standards for entry into educational programs and nursing practice and developing a common understanding of credentialing. Other key elements of a profession are a code of ethics, a basis for systematic theory development, peer review to ensure standards of practice, and a professional culture sustained by professional associations.[90-93]

Knowing these well established elements of professionalism, it is incongruous to observers that individuals and groups of nurses have not unified in defining fundamental professional goals for nursing education and practice. Testimony revealed that the lack of unity in nursing's professional goals not only causes confusion in education and practice matters, but also lowers nursing's status.

Nursing's Professional Development
Both the literature review and testimony contain many references to nursing's professional development in practice and education. The advancement of university-based education for nurses and increasing competence in care technologies have fostered a public image of nurses.[94] Certification programs, representation for nurses in specialty practice, and improved relationships with physicians in corresponding specialties were presented in testimony as positive results of the collective action of specialty nursing associations.

It also was learned in testimony that nursing as a profession lacks cohesiveness and a clear understanding of its role and direction. Although the professional society clearly has established the basis for common values and standards, there is a lack of acceptance on the part of nurses. Staff nurses testified that low membership in existing nursing organizations results from lack of responsiveness to their needs. Thus, organizations structured to meet the needs of the grass roots level nurse likely are to gain the greatest support within the profession.

Pluralism in Nursing
Nursing presents pluralistic and diverse values to the public, which may be both a strength and a weakness. An example of its strength is that nursing is perceived as a viable option for individuals from socially and economically deprived groups seeking upward mobility. Nurse aide, practical nursing, associate degree, diploma,

and baccalaureate educational programs provide diversity to accommodate students with varying amounts of academic aptitude and financial resources. These programs all lead to employment in a field in which shortages ensure placement of graduates.

An example of a weakness is lack of clarity in the identity of the nurse. Consequently, nursing's public and professional image lacks clarity.[95-97] Fragmentation in nursing's professional associations was one cause cited in testimony for this lack of clarity. Testimony indicated that a major reason for fragmentation was the difference between expectations formed during educational preparation and the reality of nursing practice. In addition, the inflammatory issue of entry to professional practice causes division. The American Nurses' Association supports two levels of nursing with the baccalaureate as the entry level to professional practice. Other nursing organizations support the present system of education in which the associate degree, diploma, and baccalaureate all lead to professional entry. Yet other nursing organizations support one level, baccalaureate education for nursing.

Nursing's Professional Associations
The diverse and numerous associations representing nursing were noted in testimony. It was stated that there ought to be some type of structural arrangement to provide linkages among these organizations for policy formulation that must be supported by all nurses. Nursing associations limited in membership by specialty, interest, and practice setting could be linked through this arrangement to determine common goals for nursing education, practice, and credentialing. Specialization was cited to be an element of nursing's developing professionalism, but there was a strong challenge for cohesive leadership in nursing's professional associations.

Many presenters in testimony challenged nursing's professional associations to be more responsive to staff nurses. Many staff nurses indicated that they did not belong to nursing associations because of high costs of time, energy, and resources needed to participate. They felt lack of support from their employers, and believed that nurses in education and in administrative positions were freer to participate. Consequently, the associations, in their view, represented educators and administrators, not staff nurses.

Credentialing
The importance of a credentialing system, supported and accepted by the profession as a whole, was cited in testimony as an essential component of professionalism, career mobility, and professional interaction. Credentialing was considered an essential element in levels of practice and clinical progression programs in ensuring

public safety and trust in specialized nursing services, and in linking the educator and clinician and the nurses and the physicians in collaborative practice.

Credentialing was viewed as central to changing the image of nursing from one controlled by institutional design to that of a professional career. Fostering the development of a leadership cadre in nursing, recognizing advanced competence through certification accepted by the profession as a whole, and compensating nurses for their increased contribution to patient care related to competence would result from a clear credentialing system, in the opinion of those presenting testimony.

Current efforts to implement recommendations of the ANA-sponsored *Study of Credentialing in Nursing* (completed in 1979) provides the profession with an opportunity to achieve the necessary consensus about this fundamental professional issue.[98-102]

Nursing and Public Policy
Public policy representatives testifying at the public hearings indicated that lacking direction from within the profession, nursing is subject to external regulation of education and practice through statutes, regulatory actions, allocation of funds, or other means.[103] It was emphasized in testimony that nursing can neither demand status nor achieve initiatives in public policy unless there is agreement within nursing about nursing's education, practice, and credentialing.

The need for nurses to act collectively through their organizations was emphasized in testimony. Collective action was viewed as creating an organized, democratic framework in which nurses promote change to improve patient care and from which nurses derive public policy initiatives and the strength to participate effectively in policy formulation for nursing and health care.

Professional Identity and Recruitment
A clear professional identity for nursing also is important in recruitment of students to nursing. In most state studies that include projections of nursing supply and demands, shortages of nurses for the 1980s and beyond are predicted.[104] A survey of 1980 high school graduates in Kentucky showed that female enrollments in professional schools such as law and medicine increased while enrollments in nursing decreased.[105] A study of projected numbers of high school graduates indicates that the numbers of graduates steadily will decline until 1985.[106]

The decrease in potential students in nursing is compounded by population changes that increase the need for nurses. The median age of the population and the number of persons over age

65 are projected to increase.[107] To meet the needs of patients in all areas of the country, it is imperative that nursing project a realistic, career-oriented image, in order to recruit successfully.

It also was emphasized in testimony that nursing effectively has not recruited men, minority members, and second-career candidates. It was suggested that nursing needs comprehensive recruitment programs targeted to diverse groups of career-oriented persons. Consensus about key issues in nursing education and practice were cited as necessary to project a clear image of the profession to attract students seeking careers.

Analysis

Fragmentation within the nursing organizations leads to a lack of clear direction for the profession. There are disagreement and confusion about the proper educational preparation for nurses, controversy about qualifications for entry to practice and lack of clarity regarding credentialing. Nurses themselves cannot agree on the desired sequence of career placement in education and practice. Lack of cohesiveness and conflicts over standards interfere with advancement of the profession and of individual nurses.

If clear direction about critical issues were provided by nursing leadership and supported by nurses in practice, nurses would be more likely to receive public recognition and support as well as improved and appropriate compensation. Deliberations within the profession and with other professional groups would be improved if nurses, differentiated by their educational preparation and credentialing mechanisms, could present clear credentials for practice.

High school graduates increasingly prepare for professions they perceive to be more rewarding than nursing. Nursing increasingly is perceived as a suitable career by upwardly mobile individuals from economically and socially disadvantaged backgrounds. There is increasing need for nurses, a declining pool of high school graduates, and a declining proportion of those graduates selecting nursing.

Recommendations

1. All of the diverse nursing constituencies must join in formulating and supporting common policies in education, credentialing, and standards for practice.
2. Credentialing mechanisms should be implemented to meet contemporary societal and professional needs with all due speed.
3. The national nursing organizations must be more in tune with and responsive to the needs of the staff nurse, including the

recognition of differences in practice settings, education, emerging specialization, and management.

4. Nurses should participate in community activities and in public policy forums about health care on a local, state, and national basis. Such efforts should be encouraged by educators and supported by employers of nurses.

5. It is the leadership responsibility of nursing organizations to implement a comprehensive recruitment program that promotes nursing as a challenging career for men, women, and persons from ethnic minority groups, and older candidates. The organizations must enlist the support of other health care organizations and academic institutions to support and disseminate accurate and current information on nursing careers to the public.

NURSES AND UNIONS;
NURSES AND SUPPLEMENTARY STAFFING AGENCIES

Retention and Recruitment

Comprehensive plans to improve nurse recruitment and retention are being developed in response to the current shortage of nurses. A comprehensive recruitment and retention program incorporates aspects of the work that nurses perform in nursing care as well as personnel policies. Such programs are considered by health care agencies to be a financial investment that employers need to protect by addressing carefully all aspects of the nurses' work and employment that affect job satisfaction.

The *Inventory of Innovative Programs and Projects* contains many examples of responses health care institutions are making to recognize nurses' needs. Types of programs underway: establishing inhouse supplementary agencies or part-time nurse pools, participating in regional supplementary agencies with other local hospitals, developing flexible scheduling patterns using 10 and 12-hour shifts or increasing staff during peak hours, and promoting systems in which staff nurses, as a group, plan their own schedules. In addition, there are child care services and loan funds for newly employed nurses with a forgiveness clause after one year of employment, and "Role Model" and "Very Important Nurse" programs. It was emphasized at the public hearings that health care institutions must examine their management practices, listen to staff nurses, and work toward comprehensive retention programs.

Factors in Nurse Satisfaction

Frequently mentioned factors that promote job satisfaction for nurses presented at the public hearings, in state studies, and in the literature review were salaries and benefits, staffing and scheduling, working conditions, and career opportunities.[108-114] In testimony, the importance of these factors was described by nurses, health care administrators, physicians, and others. When incorporated into comprehensive recruitment and retention programs, they fall into three categories: nursing roles and functions, the organizational climate in which care takes place, and personnel policies. Nurses perceived that all three were affected by the structure of health care institutions.

Nursing Roles and Functions

Nurses testified that they are more satisfied when they use their nursing abilities more fully. They expect to have decision-making authority for nursing process, defined as a sequence of assessing, planning, implementing, and evaluating nursing care according to the patient's needs and preferences and working with other health care professionals in complementary roles—especially physicians. In many organizational modes for nursing care delivery, however, nursing functions are designed as prescribed tasks to be carried out on a given schedule determined by institutional prerogatives and constraints. To nurses, having professional autonomy means exercising professional discretion over the nursing process and using institutional resources in a cost-effective manner to provide patient care.

The Organizational Climate

The organizational climate in which care takes place is influenced by the philosophy, values, and attitudes that determine relationships employees have with one another and with other health care professionals. Respect and mutual trust are two values nurses seek. Nurses expect to develop and implement care plans for patients during their hospitalization. Staffing based on slots to be filled to "cover" the unit indicated to nurses who testified that they were perceived as conventional workers rather than professionals. Being expected to perform nonnursing support services was considered by nurses to indicate lack of understanding of the value of nursing care.

Personnel Policies

Personnel policies also were thought to be indicators of underlying values and attitudes about nursing care. The expectation that nurses work days, evenings, and nights in the same week, overtime requirements, and float from one patient care area to another suggested lack of respect for and understanding of the complex demands of nursing care.

29

Some nurses mentioned other concerns related to working conditions in their testimony. Educational benefits, time off to attend professional workshops and meetings, and promotion plans based on education, experience, and competence were important to them for professional growth. Lack of opportunities for career development indicated lack of respect for their professional status. Low salaries reflected lack of respect for and understanding of essential nursing care services.

Other factors in the work environment—day care centers, availability of adequate food service, lounges, and transportation and parking facilities—were important to nurses. Provisions of these services indicated to nurses not only that they were valued employees, but that employers understood their needs and appreciated their commitment to patient care.

Nursing's Commitment

The commitment that nurses are expected to have to patient care was acknowledged in testimony. Physicians and health care administrators as well as nurse administrators depended on the commitment of staff nurses. In the state studies, nurse administrators indicated that in times of shortages, they preferred to ask their nurse employees to work extra shifts, as opposed to employing agency nurses. Nurses, on the other hand, said that commitment must be balanced with satisfaction in performance of professional nursing care in a climate that promotes professionalism and working conditions that recognize their value. A major cause of frustration cited was being asked to give more time and effort without—or for insufficient—reward.

Nurses who become frustrated with the inability to practice nursing as it should be practiced or who cannot influence their working conditions or gain improved personnel policies and benefits can choose from several options: leave nursing, seek another position in the same or different health care agency, endure their present position, seek some form of collective action, join a union, or work for a supplementary staffing agency.

Collective Action

Participation in groups by nurses in an institution or professional nursing association was reported in testimony to be effective for many. A few nurses reported lack of success with collective action, and others said the only way they could get management to listen was to become involved with third party groups who could intervene for them.

Unions

The extent to which and the conditions under which nurses select the option to have a third party represent them is not fully known. Review of the literature suggests that, following the 1974 amendment to the National Labor Relations Act, unionization of health care employees would be expected to accelerate.[114-116]

Representation by State Nurses' Associations

Historically, through state and local associations, the ANA has represented the majority of nurses who seek to be organized and represented. Trade unions increasingly are seeking registered nurses to join their ranks. Loss of membership and revenue to unions that have represented the labor force in large industries is one reason given in the literature for unions' eagerness to organize the health care field.

The ANA, however, has a long-standing history as a labor organization, registered as such in 1946 to gain improved status and working conditions for nurses. The issues of economic security, job flexibility, and improved working conditions that have led nurses to seek collective bargaining through the state nurses' associations (SNAs) historically have been the most controversial and sometimes divisive issues among the employed nurses, the professional organization, and employing agencies. Because the ANA has become a third-party representative, as well as nursing's representative of professionalism, there also is some public confusion about its true role.

Labor Organizations and Professionalism

Some nurses believe that the role of labor organizations and professionalism conflict. Those who feel this way about ANA's dual professional and labor activities question how long the organization can remain viable because of division of organizational resources. Some nurses do not belong to the ANA because it is a registered labor organization; others join but do not support its collective bargaining activities, although they support its professional activities.

Other nurses believe that labor organizations and professionalism are compatible and support the use of collective bargaining as a tool through which they can gain discretion in practice matters. In both testimony and in the literature review, some nurses reported that representation through SNAs was preferable to representation by trade unions because SNAs promote professionalism of nurses and professional health care values. Sensitivity to the professional and status concerns may, however, preclude the SNA's becoming a strong negotiator; trade unions were perceived by some to be more aggressive bargaining agents.

Nurses join unions as a mechanism to improve working conditions, salaries, and aspects of nursing practice. But some authors believe nurses should attempt to achieve these goals through professionalism. In one view, professionalism and unionism fundamentally are different; unionism tends to establish uniformity that nurses believe interferes with their decision-making authority in patient care. Professionalism, on the other hand, establishes responsibility, initiative, and merit.[120] Others view unions as an emerging mechanism to achieve professional goals, but a professional model of bargaining has yet to be developed.[121]

Motivation to Join Unions

There are few studies on nurses' motivation to join unions. Increased salaries, flexible working hours, and improved working conditions were common reasons given in most studies.[122-127] In one study, it was found that nurses who opposed unions felt that management listened to them. In another study, it was found that most of the unionized nurses worked in urban and large hospitals. Making management listen, improved salaries and benefits, grievance procedures, a way to change outdated policies and procedures, and more recognition and discretion in matters of nursing practice were findings that supported their decisions.

Effectiveness of Representation

Both testimony and literature indicate that nurses are not always satisfied with the results of joining a union. A long-term lawsuit resulting from the employer's refusal to bargain was cited in testimony; contracts resulting in fewer benefits than nurses previously had were described in the public hearings. The health care institutions' constrained fiscal resources were cited by some authors as a limitation in aggressive bargaining by unions. One author related a description of nurses' disenchantment with unions after finding that the union was not the "security blanket" that shielded them from problems.[130-132] On the other hand, nurses testified that nursing must be represented; if management is not proactive in efforts to improve the work, working environment, and personnel policies, nurses will seek unions or other options.

Supplementary Staffing Agencies

Another option for nurses is working for a supplementary staffing agency. Although nursing registries for private duty nursing have been in existence for years, new forms of supplementary agencies have proliferated. Nurses testifying at the public hearings said they chose to work for supplementary agencies because of flexible hours, choice of assignment, lack of tolerance for long hours, and conditions in their former employment. Variety in assignment and an opportunity to gain experience before seeking permanent employment are two other reasons reported in the literature.[133]

In testimony and in the literature review, it was learned that extensive use of agency nurses disrupted the quality and continuity of care. Lowered morale of permanent staff nurses also was reported.[134-135] Positive effects of supplementary agencies also were presented in testimony. Increased staffing needs during periods of high patient census, temporary replacement of nurses on vacation or leave, and interim staffing when opening new facilities were three conditions cited in which nurses from supplemental staffing agencies were found helpful to hospitals.

Analysis

Many nurses have indicated a lack of success in changing their working conditions, salaries, and autonomy in practice and seek employment with supplementary agencies or assistance through collective bargaining organizations. It is perceived that the growth of nursing unions and supplementary agencies is the result of various dissatisfactions in the work setting that nurses perceive to be related to the structure of the health care practice setting. Nurses who seek employment in supplementary agencies often cite the same motivation as those who join unions. Improved salaries, flexible schedules, and improved working conditions are three major factors behind nurses' move to supplementary agencies or unions. Many nurses join unions in an effort io improve their participation in patient care decisions and opportunities for career advancement. Other nurses do not join unions, believing that union membership is inconsistent with their professionalism.

The effects of unions on patient care and nurses' job satisfaction have not been extensively studied. Some nurses have fewer benefits after union negotiation than they had previously, while others report improved working conditions and benefits as a result of union activity.

Recommendations

1. Perceptions that the growth of nursing unions and supplementary agencies is the result of various sources of dissatisfaction in the work setting should be studied. The cause and effect of such dissatisfaction should be evaluated.

2. Employers should evaluate conditions of nurse employment to ensure an appropriate work setting, adequate salaries, flexible scheduling patterns, and nurses' involvement in clinical and institutional decision-making.

Chapter

3

NURSING EDUCATION

Efforts to increase the supply of nurses to meet recurring shortages during the past 50 years have led to several types of nursing education programs. The lack of a clearly defined structure for nursing education causes redundancy in educational costs for basic nursing, graduate, and continuing education. The associate degree, diploma, and baccalaureate programs all lead to registered nurse licensure. The transition of nursing education to a system commensurate with higher education in the United States parallels the growth of post secondary education, but has caused a marked separation between nursing practice and education.

The key relationships related to nursing education are:

A. The Nursing Profession and Education
B. Nursing Education and Nursing Practice

THE NURSING PROFESSION AND NURSING EDUCATION

The current shortage of nurses has necessitated attention to maintaining an adequate supply of nurses to meet the needs for nursing care across the nation. Many persons presenting testimony acknowledged the dependency of health care institutions on the educational system for a source of clinically competent nurses. There was strong support in testimony to support all levels of nursing education. Documented shortages of staff nurses, nurse administrators with masters degrees, clinical nurse practitioners, nurse educators, and nurse researchers were reported.

Emphasis was placed on the need for statewide planning for nursing education at all levels, basic through doctoral, for consensus among educators about appropriate linkages among educational programs, and for master plans to guide allocation of resources for nursing education.

Graduations from Nursing Schools

Data from the National League for Nursing[1] were presented in testimony and in the literature review. These data indicate that there will be a two to three-percent per year decline in registered nurse graduates through 1985. In 1979 there were 77,932 graduations from all types of registered nurse programs; the projected decline will result in 67,556 graduations in 1985. Graduations from associate degree and diploma programs were shown to have declined from 1977-78 to 1978-79 at a rate of 0.99 percent for associate degree and 0.92 percent for diploma programs. Graduations from baccalaureate nursing programs were predicted to increase slightly in 1980-81. There was an increase of 1.03 percent in baccalaureate graduations from 1978 to 1979, but a decline was predicted from 1981-85.

Reasons given for the decline in graduations from nursing programs were demographic changes, such as declining numbers of high school graduates, despite admission of more persons over the age of 21; cost containment; changing staffing patterns in health care institutions; and the impact of expanded nursing roles. These possible unknown influences may change predictions for the future supply of nurses.[2]

Registered Nurse Enrollments

The number of registered nurses returning to school for baccalaureate education has increased steadily since 1974. The increase was 68.8 percent in the North Atlantic region, 98.9 percent in the midwest, 45.9 in the Southern region, and 40.9 percent in the Western region. The average for all regions was 70.9 percent, representing a change from 3,791 registered nurses graduated in 1974-75 to 6,480 in 1978-79.[3] Of nurses licensed in 1977, 6.8 percent of associate degree graduates returned to college as compared with 9.6 percent of diploma graduates; and 12.2 percent of baccalaureate graduates enrolled in masters level programs.[4] Continuing formal education was a reason given for leaving employment in nursing in both North and South Carolina's state studies.[5]

Nursing Education in Transition

Generally, it was acknowledged in testimony that nursing education is in transition. Not only are nurses seeking to upgrade their education, but programs are undergoing transition to accommodate registered nurse students and to ensure educational mobility through the system of nursing education.

Statewide Planning

Several state studies about nursing education included plans for defining career paths through the educational system.[6] In one plan, the number of initial admissions plus the number of returning licensed practical and registered nurses advancing to the next degree were projected. The returning students were called "mobilists" and were included in estimations of funding needs for each type of nursing program. In several states, statewide planning to define competencies for graduates of associate degree, diploma, and baccalaureate programs were either completed or reported to be in progress, to promote advancement through the educational system. A clearly defined system of nursing education in some state plans was plotted in a sequence from associate, baccalaureate, masters, to doctoral programs.

Regional Planning

A number of regional and local plans for linking educational programs were presented in testimony, in the literature, and in the *Inventory of Innovative Programs and Projects*. The North Carolina Articulation Project, sponsored by the University of North Carolina and the Department of Community Colleges, is an example of projects to establish guidelines for transfer of credit. Minimum behavioral expectations of new graduates from New Mexico schools of nursing were developed as the basis for job descriptions for new graduates in various areas of clinical practice in the New Mexico statewide effort, The System for Nursing Articulation Program (SNAP).

Another articulated nursing education system includes a sequence of nursing education from vocational to doctoral levels; each level is based on a foundation of competencies in core curricula so that the components of the nursing programs are articulated.[7] Students complete designated competencies for each level and do not repeat this learning in the next level if they choose to continue their nursing education.

Need for Consensus

The majority of state studies about nursing education cited the need for a clearly defined, articulated system of nursing education.[8] Consensus among nurse educators, nurse administrators, and others was developed through task force groups or committees. Membership also included representation from boards of higher education, health care administrators, consumers, and others. It was emphasized in testimony that the process of defining the system of nursing education in the state or region required agreement about resource allocation, funding, and educational methodology. The need to plan educational sequences to prevent redundancy was emphasized in testimony.

Cost of Nursing Education

Many persons presenting testimony cited concern for financial aspects of nursing education. It was reported that the true cost of nursing education has not yet been determined. Diploma education was reported to add cost to patient care. However, in both testimony and in the literature review, hospitals with schools reported lower or similar costs per patient than those without schools.[9] The anticipated results of a National League for Nursing study of the costs of nursing education were cited to be important in sorting out nursing education costs. Educational resources in many states were reported to be constrained. Consequently, improved data about the supply and demand for nurses, relating nursing education to nursing practice, and deleting redundancy from the educational system through a clearly defined sequence of career advancement, were cited as needs in testimony, state studies, and in the literature. The responsibility for nursing education was considered by many to be a primary concern for states. Because the majority of nurse graduates tend to remain in the state where they are educated, the state's investment in nursing education is justified. About 62 percent of employed nurses were found to live in the same state where they completed their basic nursing education.[10] Of importance is the states' concern for protecting the public safety and welfare, and ensuring that the public need for nursing care will be met. Variations in types and numbers of nursing education programs within states, however, were cited in testimony and are apparent from review of state studies.

A total of 15 states have fewer than 10 nursing programs; nine states have no diploma programs and there were 114 masters level programs in 1977-78.[11] There are only 30 masters programs in nursing that offer a major in nursing administration. There are 22 doctoral programs for nursing in the United States.* State and regional variations also were found in the numbers of registered nurses available per population. It was apparent from testimony that planning for nursing education must take into account not only national accreditation, but state and regional variations in numbers and accessibility of programs.

---

* Information obtained from the American Association of Colleges of Nursing.

Reentry Programs

In some states, programs to promote reentry of nurses were conducted in response to the nursing shortage. A survey of inactive nurses was reported by the Task Force on Nursing Shortage in Virginia; of 3,480 nurses responding, 30 percent cited need for refresher course as a reason for not returning to active nursing.[12] The Indiana Commission for Higher Education reported that 13 refresher courses were provided in Indiana to attract nurses from the pool of inactive registered nurses in the state.[13] Of the 120 nurses who participated in the refresher courses, 40 percent returned to practice.

It was noted in testimony, however, that refresher programs had not proved cost-effective in some settings. A low rate of return to employment following completion of refresher courses also was reported in some state studies. It was suggested that educational opportunities to foster reentry of inactive nurses should be made part of the system of higher education. Reentry should be formalized and targeted to those who drop out of nursing during childbearing years.

Entry to Practice

Entry to practice was frequently mentioned in testimony as a factor in nursing's current educational transition. Nursing's failure to resolve the entry to professional practice issue was viewed as symbolic of the profession's future direction that now is shifting to the issue of the relationship between nursing education and practice. It generally was agreed that levels of knowledge and skill of nurse graduates need to be validated for all types of nursing education programs to ease the transition to practice and to establish a comprehensible and consistent foundation for sequential educational programs and for continuing education following graduation. The entry to practice issue was cited as an incentive for many registered nurses to enter baccalaureate nursing programs to protect their investment in their career, as well as to advance their careers. It also was cited as a factor in the movement of diploma programs to the higher education system.

Nontraditional Nursing Education

That nursing education is in transition was acknowledged in testimony. A trend in this transition phase was reported to be development of nontraditional programs. Models presented in testimony demonstrate the effectiveness of nontraditional nursing education. It was emphasized that these programs must meet criteria of sound academic principles. Acceptance of programs that vary from the norm by nurse educators and accreditation groups was reported to be uneven.

Gaining acceptance by accreditation groups was a common problem cited in testimony by many persons involved in nontraditional educational programs. Reevaluation of accreditation criteria to determine guidelines to promote quality in nontraditional nursing education commensurate with academic standards in the system of higher education was urged. The extent to which current accreditation criteria encourage or discourage development of nontraditional nursing programs has not been studied extensively. A few persons who reported development of innovative hospital-college arrangements said they had received state approval and accreditation from the regional accreditation body for higher education.

Resources for Nursing Education

The need to use educational resources effectively and to recognize the clinical resources of health care institutions were cited in testimony. The trend toward upper division nursing courses in baccalaureate programs and the ability of health care institutions to serve as the clinical resource for the nursing component of baccalaureate programs were emphasized in the rationale to establish baccalaureate education in settings previously used for diploma education.

Another trend reported was development of models for transition of diploma education to the system for higher education. Several options for programs were offered. Some diploma schools have become or are becoming degree granting institutions. Others have contracted with local colleges or universities to establish baccalaureate nursing education programs through shared resources. Examples of these options are in the *Inventory of Innovative Programs and Projects.*

Educational Opportunities for Registered Nurses

Several examples of flexible programs designed to meet the special needs of registered nurse students were presented in testimony and in the literature, and the *Inventory of Innovative Programs and Projects.* The Colorado State Nurses' Association described the Butterfly Project to bring baccalaureate nursing educators together to share information and support for registered nurses seeking upward mobility. Diverse educational needs of registered nurses are being met by innovations in educational methodology and by flexible weekend and evening course schedules. Individualized programs based on mastery learning concepts, credit by challenge examinations, and other methods were reported in the literature, testimony, and the *Inventory of Innovative Programs and Projects.* A masters level program that builds on associate degree and diploma program curricula and promotes educational advancement without redundancy also was described.[14]

Accessibility of Education

In testimony, opportunities for continuing formal education were cited as important to nurses. This finding was documented in many state studies. A few staff nurses reported that they received credit for their nursing education in other fields, completed degrees, and had achieved successful second careers. Typical of these nurses' testimony was a feeling of frustration about not receiving credit for previous nursing education in a baccalaureate nursing program, but also a feeling of satisfaction with their present achievement.

Other staff nurses reported positive experiences in completing baccalaureate nursing programs, saying they received credit for competence they had achieved, that the program had expanded and updated their professional competence, and that they provided better patient care as a result.

Nursing education is supported by many health care institutions. Scholarship and loan programs, reimbursement for education, and other forms of educational support were reported in testimony. Involvement of health care auxilians and community groups in providing financial support for nursing education was reported at the Open Forums for Small and Rural Hospitals, held by the American Hospital Association's Center for Small or Rural Hospitals. Work/[15] study programs and support for program development also were cited in testimony and in the open forums.

Nursing as a Career

Action directed to developing a clear direction for nursing education should foster recruitment of students into nursing. Because societal values promote careers for women, nursing must develop an educational system commensurate with the system of higher education in the United States.

Potential students need to be able to examine their options for career choices according to the generally accepted meanings of different levels of education. It was stated in testimony that the possibilities for career advancement through graduate and higher degrees in nursing should be clearly defined and as accessible as those in other professional fields. These same options should be accessible to registered nurses who desire advanced education. Many who presented testimony felt that clearly defined career paths through the educational system were essential to ensure that the shortages of nurses at all levels of education projected for the 1980s and beyond would not occur.

41

Analysis

The existence of several types of nursing education that lead to registered nurse licensure—mainly associate degree, diploma, and baccalaureate—has engendered debate and controversy about educational requirements for practice. The major debate focuses on the proposal that the baccalaureate degree be viewed as the minimum requirement for entry to professional practice. Nurses who wish to upgrade their education perceive lack of opportunity. The nursing profession will be enhanced if nursing agrees on and implements a clear system of nursing education that promotes realistic expectations and provides appropriate support for practice and advancement.

Recommendations

1. Educational mobility in nursing for undergraduate and registered nurses must be promoted in the higher education system (baccalaureate) through educational articulation between components of the educational system. Programs should be accessible. Special programs for successful reentry of nurses should be developed.
2. Baccalaureate education for professional nursing practice is a desirable goal. In achieving this goal, consideration must be given to regional differences in availability of educational programs, educational funds, practice settings, available faculty, and potential students.
3. Existing private and public funds supporting nursing education should be preserved. Nursing education resources should be allocated to ensure adequate numbers of nurses in basic and graduate programs for clinical practice, education, research, and administration.
4. Accreditation standards should encourage an articulated education system in nursing. The perception that accreditation requirements encourage or discourage innovations in education and career mobility should be studied and appropriately modified.

NURSING PRACTICE AND NURSING EDUCATION

The strongest investment nursing can make in its future is to resolve the debate between nursing education and nursing practice. At the public hearings, the fundamental goals of nursing education were acknowledged: prepare clinically competent nurses who can function as full members of the patient care team; maintain high standards of professional nursing practice; and ensure high quality of nursing care. It also was acknowledged that the patient care environment has increased in complexity due to clinical advances in health care technology and the emergence of new organizational modes for nursing care delivery. Nurses are seeking a sequence of education and a nursing practice that offers career advancement.

Historical causes of the schism between nursing education and practice presented in testimony and in the literature stem from changes both in nursing education and practice. Movement of nursing education from hospitals to the system of higher education began the alienation that is just beginning to be confronted.[16]

Nurse Educators' Perspective

Many nurse educators believe in the traditional focus on liberal arts learning, unifying the purpose of collegiate nursing education, and individual and social benefits of college education for a meaningful life.[17] Nurse educators have had to enter the debate between the academic purists and pragmatists about the nature and purpose of college education. Nursing education, because it prepares graduates for work, is considered pragmatic. Establishing nursing as a legitimate academic field of study in colleges and universities has necessitated overcoming resistance from purists.

Employers' Perspective

In testimony, employers of nurses stated their goals for nursing education: graduates who are clinically competent to carry out patient care responsibilities; clinically competent nursing faculty; curricula in nursing schools attuned to the changing and real world of nursing; and students prepared for the intensity and acuity of patient needs, who are socialized to desired behaviors of practicing nurses, and who are committed to nursing. Adequate clinical experience, continuity in clinical experience, and emphasis on care of acute patients were considered important by many in testimony.

Economic Constraints

Despite their different missions, education and practice institutions face similar economic constraints. Resources for education, in general, are shrinking. Increased costs and decreasing sources of funding for nursing education were cited in testimony and by many authors.[18-19] Schools have been challenged to reduce the cost per student by accelerating programs, re-examining the faculty teaching role, using off-campus alternatives, establishing consortia among institutions, and other methods.

Equally constraining are cost containment imperatives in health care institutions. Cost-effectiveness defined as utilizing the minimum resources required to produce desired results is a component of every nurse adminstrator's function. Extensive program evaluation methodology that nurse administrators must incorporate for every activity was described in the literature.[20] Nurse administrators not only must develop cost-effective structures for care delivery, but for the functions needed, such as education to support nurses in their professional growth.

Elimination of Redundancy
One of the important reasons for developing a clear sequence of nursing education and practice is elimination of redundancy of effort and cost between the two. Currently, nursing education provides a wide range of educational programming, including preparation in basic, graduate, and continuing education. Health care institutions also provide a wide range of educational programs; orientation, staff development, and continuing education are part of many health care institutional programs. Some health care institutions, according to both testimony at the public hearings and the Open Forums for Small and Rural Hospitals, do not have the educational resources required, and cannot afford to acquire them.

Education in Health Care Institutions
The expanded educational component of nursing management units has grown for several reasons. It was reported in testimony that the nurses' need for extensive orientation as well as the trend toward mandatory or voluntary continuing education have required increased attention to education in practice settings. Another important reason was the acknowledged link between educational programs and the quality of nursing care. Educational interventions are one method used to rectify deficits in patient care, revealed by audit, to assure the desired quality of care.[21-22]

That health care institutions have assumed an increasing role and cost in educating nurses is evidenced by the escalating costs of orientation. In 1974, the average cost of orienting one nurse in a hospital of 500-plus beds was approximately $900.[23] In a recent study conducted in a 300-bed hospital, orientation costs for each new nurse averaged $1685.[24]

Not only have orientation efforts been expanded in practice settings, but staff development has expanded. The lack of distinction between staff development and continuing education was reported in testimony. Both are included in most educational programs in larger hospitals and they often overlap. The nurse administrator, in developing and implementing these programs, must have budget

44

and qualified staff, and must express the philosophy for care in the institution.[25-30]

Lack of qualified faculty was cited in testimony as a problem by some nurse administrators as was lack of adequate budget. Some institutions, particularly small and rural hospitals, have few resources to devote to educational functions.[31] The sophisticated programs described in the literature are beyond the reach of nurses in these institutions.[32-35]

Defining Competencies

A well defined trend emerging from the state studies, literature review, and testimony was defining competencies of nurse graduates. The clear differentiation among the three types of basic nursing education programs—associate, diploma, and baccalaureate—ceases once the nurse begins employment, but is maintained in educational settings.

Competency levels of nurses are being studied in several states to provide improved career mobility through education for registered nurses. Nurse educators and many nurses in clinical practice cited the need to differentiate in employment the job expectations and salaries for nurses according to types of basic programs.

Health care administrators, public policy representatives, and others challenged nursing to examine its programs. If there really are differences in competencies of graduates from each type of program, nursing must rethink its scheme of employing, at the same salaries and in the same positions, the three types of graduates.

On the other hand, if there are no differences among associate degree, diploma, and baccalaureate programs, with regard to clinical preparation and practice competency, nursing must rethink its position about education.

In a time of economic constraint, public policy representatives, in testimony, questioned what type of program can produce needed competencies of graduates for the least cost, and how many graduates are needed from the various types of programs to provide the level of patient care necessary to ensure public safety and welfare.

Performance of Registered Nurses

The ambiguities in the current relationship between nursing education and practice were discussed in testimony and literature. It generally was agreed that because of the lack of clear differentiation in competency levels of graduates, the performance of nurses is more dependent on the personal characteristics of students, their level of academic scholarship, and the demands and characteristics of the practice setting, regardless of type of education program.

Organizational structure for nursing care delivery, leadership, and staff morale also were cited as features of the practice setting that influence performance of registered nurses.

Several researchers have studied the performance of graduates from different types of nursing education programs. Bassett found no significant difference in the creative thinking ability and problem-solving skill between baccalaureate and associate degree graduates.[36] Frederickson and Mayer found no difference in the process used by baccalaureate and associate degree students to solve problems.[37] Gray, however, found that associate degree graduates concentrated more on patients' immediate needs and baccalaureate graduates concentrated more on their long-term needs.[38] Bullough and Sparks found that baccalaureate and associate degree nurses differ in orientation to patient care, a difference related to the technical orientation of faculty.[39] These results suggest that, although students from different types of programs appear to use the same process, the focus of each type of program differs.

Petti found no conclusive differences among diploma, associate, and baccalaureate graduates.[40] Nelson, however, found that baccalaureate graduates were rated higher by supervisors, but diploma graduates rated higher in technical and administrative skills and baccalaureate graduates rated higher in communication skills.[41] Davis found that the quality and quantity of patient care improved with increasing education, and was highest for clinical specialists with masters degrees.[42]

The high pass-rate on state board examinations by diploma graduates was reported in testimony at the public hearings. Behm and Warnock, however, compared performance on state boards and the effectiveness of associate degree programs.[43] There was a small but not significant relationship. These authors concluded that state board examinations were not predictors of how students perform in practice. Knopf found that baccalaureate graduates tended to assume teaching and administrative roles more frequently than did diploma or associate degree graduates.[44]

Need for Clarity in Education
In testimony, presenters indicated that differences among basic educational programs were of strategic importance in attracting career-oriented students to nursing. The perceived dissonance between types of education and nursing practice, which has not been substantiated in research or in observation, was reported to adversely affect nursing's public image and recruitment of students into nursing.

In the current climate of economic constraint, and of decreasing graduations from nursing programs, the viability of the current pluralistic system of nursing education was questioned. The cost of the debate between nursing education and service also is reflected in disillusionment of new graduates, leading to increased turnover and, for some, career drop-out.[45-47]

Nursing thus was challenged at the public hearings to rationalize its systems of education and practice. This recurring theme also is substantiated in the literature. Montag wrote, "There might be less role ambiguity and debate today if programs and requirements for technical and professional practice had been spelled out in the beginning.[48] A simpler curricular approach would result in two kinds of nurses and two kinds of programs. This simplified system of education could be carried through to the practice setting with different job descriptions, according to educational preparation, and different salary structures, according to the amount of responsibility for each. Other authors agreed that there should be two levels of personnel; those prepared at the baccalaureate level would be nurses and those prepared at the technical level would be given another title.[49]

Changing Education—Practice Relationships

Another strong theme voiced in testimony at the public hearings was the need to restructure the relationship between practice and education through cooperative efforts of educators and nurses in practice. Some held that current and real constraints in the amount of clinical practice in all types of health professional schools, not just nursing, required cooperative efforts to develop a new and rational sequence of education, planned transition, career advancement in practice, and continuing education. In this process, both curricula in schools of nursing and the structure of nursing practice in practice settings would have to be changed.

Findings of one research effort indicated that nursing roles and functions are not always explained and not consistently valued in the practice setting.[50] However, several programs aimed at improving communication between nursing education and nursing practice were outlined in testimony and in the *Inventory of Innovative Programs and Projects.* The Hahn Foundation Nursing Project and the Southeast Ohio Nursing Education-Service Consortium are two examples of regional groups of nurse educators and nursing service administrators working together to implement cooperative solutions to practice and education-related problems.[51] In another instance, a demonstration project is underway to ease transition through joint development of sequential education and orientation competencies between participating educational programs and health care institutions.[52]

Better coordination of curriculum requirements and expectations in the practice setting also was described in the literature. Examples are changing curriculum to include relevant nursing care plans, discharge planning, and patient teaching, so that students would learn competencies appropriate to the practice setting[53] and curriculum changes developed to improve the practice competencies of graduates.[54-55] Other authors described how changing the delivery system to a primary nursing care mode necessitated revising the leadership course for nursing students.[56]

Transition Programs

A number of transition programs for new graduates were described in testimony and in the literature. Internship programs were defined as extended orientation programs in which clinical experience is supplemented with discussion groups and instructional sessions. Coco evaluated internship programs ranging from 10 weeks to one year and found that these programs resulted in 63-100 percent retention for one year.[57] Coco asserted that the effects of internships should be evaluated over the long run.

A number of externship programs are reported in the *Inventory of Innovative Programs and Projects,* in which nursing students participate in guided learning experiences for the summer. Educational objectives are evaluated and students receive college credit for participation.

Other programs designed to ease the transition of new graduates into practice were reported. One example is bicultural training programs intended to reduce attrition.[58] Cost-savings resulting from this program were evaluated, and it was found that of 31 percent of the nurses who resigned in 1977, 28 percent had not participated in the workshops, whereas 3 percent had completed the entire program. Interaction modeling was used in another setting to aid new graduates to develop team leading skills.[59]

In one institution, nurse mentors provided new graduates with assistance. The mentor teaches, counsels, coaches, supports, and promotes team members.[60] Preceptor roles were described as effective, but because the concept is new, educational programs must be conducted for preceptors, if they are to be effective.

Orientation programs tailored to individuals with different levels of competency were described in the literature. One report was of an experimental competency-based orientation program in which this approach was more cost-effective than the traditional program.[61] The program lasted from two to six weeks, with an average participation of 3.2 weeks.

RESTRUCTURING FACULTY ROLES

The clinical expertise of faculty was frequently mentioned in the public hearings. Emerging forms of faculty participation in clinical practice were found both in testimony and in the literature review. Three types of faculty arrangements, designed to achieve better balance in the professional roles of education, practice, and research, were explained in one report.[62] Christman's unification model was described as the practitioner-teacher appointment that emphasizes clinical expertise. A second model of joint appointment involves joint reimbursement and establishment of separate role identities in two institutions. In a third model, faculty members arrange clinical practice positions on their own. A system is suggested for earning continuing education credits by faculty who achieve the full professional role for service, education, consultation, and research.

A method of using faculty contracts to monitor faculty performance in the full professional role in education and practice activities is described by other authors.[63] Lack of published research about how to achieve the optimal balance among the service, teaching, and research roles of professionals also was reported in the literature.[64] Affiliations are being established that incorporate clinical training and joint appointments for faculty, in attempts to achieve this balance.[65]

RELATING EDUCATION TO PRACTICE

Restructuring the organizational structures for nursing care delivery was another trend reported in testimony as being essential to improving relationships between nursing practice and education. The realities of the practice setting presented in testimony were that nursing is a 24-hour accountability; and available staff includes nurse aides, licensed practical nurses, and registered nurses from three different types of educational programs, and a few nurses with masters degrees in clinical specialties. The expediency of providing adequate staff, wide variations in accessibility of educational programs in different areas of the country, and demands to relate staffing to both quantifiable measures and quality patient care were cited as real and practical problems of nurse administrators.

These nurse administrators urged educators to be more responsive to their immediate needs. Arranging student clinical experiences on the evening and night shifts to improve practice readiness of student nurses was a suggestion frequently offered in testimony. Another suggestion was defining common criteria, standards, and norms for nursing care across the country, to develop a common base for evaluation of the quality of patient care. Several authors cited this need as well. Bloch, for example, emphasized the need to develop common definitions that are of practical value for measuring the quality of patient care in the practice setting.[66] These definitions also could be applied in curriculum development in schools.

Many nurse administrators cited difficulty in implementing some of the emerging organizational modes of nursing care delivery, such as primary nursing care because of the limitations in available mix of staff. They emphasized that the organizational structure for nursing care delivery must be related to the supply of nurses.

It was acknowledged that educational programs cannot prepare graduates to function in all types of organizational modes because, although they are defined as distinctly different, variants in each exist. This finding was substantiated in the literature review. Young found that there are few pure forms of the major types of defined organizational modes for functional, team, or primary nursing care in operation.[67]

The nurse administrators from hospitals that have few registered nurses and limited resources for orientation and education cited the difficulties of new graduates who were expected to manage care given by licensed practical nurses and nurse aides. These new graduates found actual practice different from their expectations.

Clinical Experience for Students
The amount of clinical practice experience in the basic nursing education program also was discussed in relation to the quality of nursing care provided in the practice setting. One author highlights the value of clinical experience in a discussion of curriculum and suggests that the value of patient care experiences preserved in the curriculum of some diploma schools should be reexamined by all types of nursing programs.[68] Health care administrators and nurses in clinical practice who voiced similar concerns in testimony also cited the need for adequate clinical experience for nurses at the masters level to provide leadership for new graduates. A system of career advancement for registered nurses also was suggested as a possible solution for providing assistance to new graduates.

Quality in Care Delivery
Streamlining the system of education and practice was proposed as a way to begin the processes of equating quality standards for nurs-

ing care to organizational modes of nursing care delivery. Because of differences in availability of types of nursing staff, a number of different organizational structures would be required. The best mix of nursing staff for each should be evaluated for outcomes of nurse satisfaction and quality of patient care. It was emphasized in testimony that the reality of economic constraints is that the level of quality must also be affordable.

Comprehensive Reorganization of the Management Unit

A comprehensive reorganization of the nursing management unit was described in the literature.[69] A framework was used to unify the fragmented components of a nursing department into an integrated unit. Quality of patient care, cost containment, patient classification systems, nursing behaviors, documents needed for the care system's organizational structures for information processes supporting care, and documentation of outcomes were integrated into the framework.

Several comprehensive programs for restructuring the management unit also were described in testimony. One nurse administrator described improved quality of care and nurse satisfaction in a system staffed with all registered nurses. Costs were the same or lower when compared with similar sized hospitals in the same area. A health care administrator described a system in which roles and functions of nurses were restructured and the organizational support redesigned. In another health care institution, a system of participative management was instituted to develop new programs and projects to improve nursing care and patient satisfaction.

Centers for Professional Interchange

Certain health care institutions have unique situations that preclude many of the innovations possible in large medical centers. At the Open Forums, held by the AHA Center for Small or Rural Hospitals, the nurses' roles were described as similar to those in small businesses in which each employee completes a variety of functions, because the total number of employees needed to care for the number of patients precludes specialization.[70] It was cited that limited resources for education stimulate a need to form alliances with larger medical centers to promote exchange of nursing expertise. Nurses from small and rural hospitals could go to the larger centers to learn new care technology. Nurses from the larger centers could go to the small hospitals to learn more about continuity of care and the scope of services offered in these settings.

This type of professional interchange was cited to depend on the establishment of norms for nursing across the country. A universal base, or core curriculum for nursing education, and a defined sequence of career advancement in practice in the country, would open the way for ongoing interchange among nurses in different settings. This sequence should be relevant to patient care in small and rural hospitals, in community hospitals located in small, middle, and large size cities, and in medical centers.

Differences in care, related to different missions of health care institutions, should be recognized, but could be developed from a common base. It was stated that all nurses should begin to understand and appreciate the value of professional communication and learning from one another across practice settings. The literature review contains references to these concepts as well. Smith reports the results of a successful experimental program conducted by a college in which students received clinical education in a rural hospital.[71] Interchange among nursing personnel from different types of health care institutions of different sizes and missions was considered to result in improved care by reducing the influence of the practice setting that now prevails through increasing professional communication.[72]

Continuing Education

Another benefit to be derived from cooperative programming among educational and health care institutions would be a more rational system for continuing education. It was cited in testimony that establishing a baseline of competency for graduates from each type of nursing program would produce cost-savings for both educational and practice settings, because orientation, staff development, and continuing education programs could be developed from this foundation.

The need to teach some new graduates competencies that others have achieved could be deleted or significantly reduced by cooperative planning, thus improving the new graduates' feeling of achievement as well as making the maximum use of available educational resources. The "lost opportunity" cost described by del Bueno,[73] would be eliminated. This cost is incurred when staff development personnel are consumed with orientation of new graduates and therefore are not available to provide educational opportunities for other nursing staff.

It was acknowledged in testimony that health care institutions have a role and responsibility for sharing in continuing education efforts essential to maintaining competency. Scarce resources for continuing education, such as lack of qualified faculty in every setting, necessitates the combining of available resources.

Many projects and programs for making continuing education accessible to nurses were described in testimony and in the *Inventory of Innovative Programs and Projects.* The Telnet Program in Georgia, the WINs program in Wisconsin, the study of continuing education in New England, and the AHEC effort in North Carolina were provided as examples of statewide and regional programs designed to improve continuing education opportunities for nurses in a wide variety of practice settings.

Improved quality of educational offerings resulted from the extensive planning processes to assess needs and develop programs relevant to nurses in practice. The goal of these programs is to improve patient care and to improve nurse satisfaction.

Colleges and universities, because of their educational resources, were urged to take the lead in designing outreach programs to meet continuing education needs of nurses through cost-effective programs. Shared facilities, use of technology, combinations of resources, and other mechanisms were suggested to improve accessibility of continuing education for nurses in practice.

Analysis

In the professions that serve patients there frequently is the perception that new graduates lack the ability immediately to perform successfully in the practice setting. Accordingly, there is the perception that new nursing graduates are not prepared immediately to function as professionals in the practice settings. Differences within and among the three basic nursing education programs and lack of differentiation in employment of the graduates of the three programs—associate degree, diploma, and baccalaureate—lead to misutilization and often underutilization of registered nurses and confusion and conflict between education and practice. Lack of communication and consensus between nursing educators and practitioners have led to inconsistency in education and practice standards, and redundancy in effort and cost. Extensive variation in orientation and transition programs for new graduates is another reflection of redundancy between practice and educational settings.

Definition of continuing education in nursing is confounded by the multiple system of education. There is no common base on which continuing education can be built. Blurring of staff development and continuing education leads to redundancy in educational efforts within health care agencies and between these agencies and educational institutions.

Recommendations

1. Appropriate utilization of nurses should be related to the competency obtained in the educational program. There must be common understanding and recognition of the different levels of competence from the different programs. There is need to develop and test education and practice models relating levels of education to clinical competencies.
2. To provide adequate clinical education for nursing students, strong affiliations between academic institutions and practice settings must be developed. Faculty in academic institutions should maintain clinical expertise and should share a common knowledge base for the development of nursing education, practice, and research.
3. Collaborative relationships should be established between colleges and universities and practice agencies for the purpose of developing continuing education. Ensuring nurses' participation in continuing education is a shared responsibility of individual nurses and employers, and local educational institutions.

Chapter

4

NURSING AND THE PUBLIC

The several facets of nursing's relationship to the public were presented in testimony at the commission's public hearings. Levels of public awareness and expectation, nurses' involvement in public policy formation for health care, state and national concern for health manpower planning, and mechanisms to ensure public safety and welfare through credentialing were discussed. Underlying all of these facets are the nature and value of the public service that nursing provides. Awareness of this service has been heightened by the nursing shortage, as reflected in numerous recent newspaper and magazine articles about nursing as well as television and radio coverage.

The Nursing Resource

State studies not only document the nursing shortage but the need for planning to ensure an adequate nursing resource. State master plans for nursing education have been developed in many states. Projection models to determine nursing supply and demand are being developed and refined to obtain realistic data that can be used for resource allocation for nursing education. Many state studies indicate the need for improved data and supply and demand models. The need for data also was emphasized by public policy representatives in their testimony at the public hearings.

Western Interstate Commission for Higher Education made projections for 1982 that indicated shortages of nurses, particularly at the bachelor and higher degree levels. Projections for nursing needs in most other state studies reviewed were similar and resulted in statewide plans for making baccalaureate and higher degree programs more accessible to registered nurses as well as increasing baccalaureate enrollments for generic nursing students. In a few states, shortages of licensed practical nurses were projected. Career mobility for licensed practical nurses to increase numbers of registered nurses was reported to be a need in many state studies and in testimony at the public hearings.

Public Awareness and Expectations

Two issues raised in the public hearings and in the literature were the levels of public awareness and expectation of nurses. A strong national public relations campaign was urged in testimony to educate the public about current nursing roles and functions. It was reported that nurses have tended to concentrate their efforts on patient care without sufficient attention to informing the public about their actual roles. The public perception of nurses' role was said to be influenced by the media's portrayal of nursing in overly dramatic images that do not reflect accurately the level of education and skill held by many nurses in practice.

Nurses' Involvement in Public Policy

In testimony, nurses were encouraged to better realize their potential to participate in public policy about health care. The expertise of nurses should be used in developing public policy about health care. It was acknowledged that nurses increasingly are becoming involved in national committees and in forums for state and national policy and decision-making about health care delivery. Nurses were urged to participate more in health care legislative activities because they not only have valuable ideas to offer, but they need to heighten public awareness of their professional status.

Use of Nursing Manpower

Nurse administrators manage million-dollar budgets and are accountable for effective use of the nursing resource. These nurses become aware of health manpower because of the demands of their roles in health care institutions. They are concerned, as are health care administrators, about state and national initiatives to ensure an adequate nursing resource. Efforts to match sufficient numbers of nurses with appropriate education to different functions required by patients in the health care system were reported in testimony, state studies, and the literature to be a priority in planning for the nursing resource.

One part of this effort is directed toward finding ways to provide the necessary patient care with the available nurses. The other part is directed toward state and national policy that influences nursing education and practice. Nurse administrators and others cited the need to identify factors that influence nurse employment. The usual economic supply and demand explanations for manpower do not seem to apply to nursing. A better understanding is needed to explain the relation between educational institutions' supply efforts and health care institutions' demand for nurses. An important aspect of this supply and demand is management of the nursing resource. Strong emphasis was given in testimony to the need to better prepare nurse administrators for this task. Complicated institutional relationships and traditional organizational structures must be evaluated and changed, if better use of the nursing resource is to be realized. Underutilization of some nurses and misutilization of others were considered to result from lack of differentiation in functions for nurses with different levels of education, a historic phenomenon in nursing services that requires current analysis as well as expert management by nurse administrators.

This analysis should be conducted to determine the competency and quality of care desired in today's health care system. Testimony about nursing competency also stressed the integral nature of nursing care in the provision of care within health care institutions. Combined medical and nursing audits were reported in testimony to be a measure of quality care that reflects the integration of medical and nursing's plan of care.

Licensure
An essential element in the health care institution's provision of high quality care was presented in testimony and in the literature review to be the assurance of the nurses' competence. Employers depend on credentials, such as licensure, to ensure the competence of new employees. Designed to protect the public safety and welfare, licensure in most states requires completion of a state-approved educational program and passing the state board examination for nursing. Accreditation standards ensure quality of educational preparation in schools; in nursing, these standards are set and implemented nationally. Licensure ensures adequacy of competency of individuals. In nursing, there is a national state board examination and each state sets its own licensure requirements. There is variation among states; in addition to basic licensure requirements, many states also have set standards for expanded nursing roles that require advanced education and certification.

All except one state uses the national state board examination for nursing as the licensure examination. The importance of maintaining this national standard was cited in testimony and in state studies as a means to facilitate the flow of the nurse workforce between the states.

The Public Health Service Subcommittee on Health Manpower Credentialing in 1977 recommended that national standards for credentialing health manpower should be developed and continually evaluated to be used for licensure, employment in the private sector and civil service, and for reimbursement.* Comprehensive standards that could be universally applied were recommended. Professional organizations, representatives in the private sector, and state governments should play a significant role in setting these national standards, with professions having a major role. State governments then could use the national uniform standards in their licensure function. Licensure as a legal and public process must ensure qualifications for practice. It was recommended that this external control be designed to protect the public and be sound and valid as to ensure effective and safe practice.

Analysis

Although nurses comprise the largest group of health care professionals, they are not always distinguished from other health professionals by patients and the public. The contribution that nurses can make toward improving health care is just beginning to be realized; nurses have not availed themselves of the opportunity to influence public policy.

Public policy initiatives for development of educational resources are complex and often nonproductive. Supply and demand models used for resource allocation by state and federal agencies are based on arbitrary numbers needed from different educational programs rather than on competencies required to meet actual patient needs.

The capability of nurses to provide primary health care increasingly is being recognized, especially in underserved areas such as inner cities, rural areas, and in small hospitals. Licensure standards are being challenged by segments of the public as to their appropriateness, thus jeopardizing uniformity and mobility. Nursing is in the early stages of development of specialty practice; the contribution that nurses can make toward improving health care is just beginning to be realized.

*Department of Health, Education, and Welfare. *Credentialing Health Manpower,* DHEW Pub. No. (OS) 77-50057, July 1977.

Recommendations

1. Nationally accepted standards for licensure must be implemented and maintained.
2. Federal funding for nursing should be targeted to demonstrate effective education and practice models that, widely disseminated, could provide the base for improved utilization and retention of nurses in the health care system.

Chapter

5

ACTION PLANS

The National Commission on Nursing, charged with developing and implementing action plans for the future, has concentrated its first year's efforts on establishing the forum necessary to achieve consensus about nursing-related issues and problems, and on collection of data and information. Commission public hearings, held in six major cities throughout the country, open forums, held in conjunction with the AHA Center for Small or Rural Hospitals, review of state studies, policy documents and the nursing literature, and a commission *Inventory of Innovative Programs and Projects* provided material for the commission's deliberations.

Information on how individuals, institutions, and organizations working together can act to resolve current nursing-related problems was examined. The preliminary recommendations were developed from these ideas. Action plans that reflect these recommendations were formed to indicate a direction that can be taken by nurses, physicians, health care administrators, researchers, representatives of professional health-related associations, and others. Areas in which action can be taken now, those that require demonstration and further study, and research questions have been compiled.

In deliberating about preliminary recommendations and initial action plans, the commission has been aware that the issues surrounding nursing cannot be resolved quickly. Correcting the shortage of nurses must involve both immediate actions to resolve immediate problems and long-term plans to deal with the deeper and often historical issues. The initial action plans reflect the commission's early direction. Its data collection activities will continue with particular attention to current ideas from those involved in health care. By sharing this information as it is received, the commission hopes to open up communication among health professionals and others and to stimulate action by individuals, groups, organizations, and others concerned with health care.

The action plans included in this report are necessarily broad and are limited to areas that appear to be of most value in improving the nursing situation in the long run. They are designed to provide direction in an environment of rapid change and development in health care. Further discussion and deliberation by the commission and groups like the commission, meeting at the local, state, and national levels, are necessary to resolve basic issues in nursing education, nursing practice, and public policy. The commission's initial action plans provide content for this discussion and deliberation.

NURSES AND PHYSICIANS;
NURSES AND HEALTH CARE ADMINISTRATORS

Immediate Goals
1. Trustees and health care administrators need to:
   - examine the organizational structure to ensure that nurse administrators are part of the policy-making bodies of the institution; have authority to collaborate on an equal footing with the medical leaders in the institution, and are qualified by education and experience.
   - promote and support complementary practice between nurses and physicians.
2. Educators of health care professionals need to:
   - examine curricula and socialization processes to ensure that collaborative approaches to planning, implementing, and evaluating patient care are developed and maintained.

Demonstration Projects
1. Consensus Groups could be formed to bring nurses, health care administrators, and physicians together to reach consensus about future goals and strategies to improve relationships, organizational practices, and patient care.
2. Management Training Centers could be established to offer short-term, intensive courses for nurses, health care administrators, physicians, and others who need management skills in health care institutions, with the intent that once established, the centers could become self-supporting. Centers should be accessible, developed from existing resources and expertise, and

located in major health care centers with cooperative university affiliations.

3. Models of new structures for nursing management units in health care institutions could be located or developed for evaluation of factors influencing their effects on nursing performance and job satisfaction. Those selected for evaluation should be designed to support the development of a more professional nursing organization that promotes:

- greater participation of nurses in institutional policy decisions related to patient care.
- nursing's self-direction and responsibility for patient care in design of nursing care delivery, and discretion in the content and terms of nursing functions.

4. Models of structures in health care institutions that facilitate conflict-resolution and communication to improve relationships among nurses, physicians, and health care administrators could be developed and/or evaluated.

Research Projects
Research is needed to determine under what conditions multidisciplinary health care teams function efficiently and effectively.

NURSES AND HEALTH CARE INSTITUTIONS

Immediate Goals
1. Health care administrators and nursing administrators together need to examine the structure of nursing as a management unit in the health care institution to:

- include nurse-administrator participation in management-board of trustees committees
- facilitate staff nurse participation in developing and evaluating personnel policies, promotion systems, benefits, staffing related to care delivery modes, support services, and working conditions
- develop career advancement programs for nurses based on clinical competencies, education, and contribution to patient care
- ensure opportunities for nurses to pursue professional development activities
- establish cost-effective organizational modes for nursing care delivery to ensure quality patient care and appropriate use of nursing competencies
- establish support systems for nonnursing functions on a 24-hour basis

- establish a climate and support for implementation of standards of practice set by the nursing profession, peer review, and self discipline
2. Nurses in practice should work collaboratively with other health care professionals in care delivery systems to:
   - participate in developing organizational structures that provide nursing involvement in policy decisions and patient care decisions related to nursing
   - determine organizational mechanisms that support professional practice, improved communication with other health professionals, and innovation to improve patient care
   - participate in setting standards for support systems for nonnursing patient care-related functions
   - promote involvement in personnel policies, staffing and scheduling policies, and wage and benefit structures to meet needs of practicing nurses
3. Educational Institutions need to develop statewide or regional educational programs for practicing nurse administrators to improve or maintain management skills. Consideration should be given to providing these programs for academic credit toward graduate degrees in nursing.

Demonstration Projects
1. Models of nursing care delivery, contrasting the costs and benefits of different combinations of staffing arrangements and personnel mix, need to be developed and/or evaluated. Models should identify organizational modes and combinations of educational background of nurses and types of patient care needs that promote quality of patient care, nurse satisfaction, and cost-effectiveness.
2. Models of career advancement systems for nurses in health care institutions need to be developed and/or evaluated. Models should demonstrate advancement in clinical, administrative, education, and research components of professional nursing roles and should link incentives to advances in education, competence, and accountability. Costs, benefits, quality of patient care, and the effects of clinical advancement programs on nursing performance and satisfaction should be evaluated.
3. Models of organizational design for nursing management units that provide mechanisms for nurse participation in clinical and managerial decisions need to be developed and/or evaluated for their impact on quality of care and nurse satisfaction.
4. Models of graduate nursing programs should be developed and/or evaluated to provide graduate degrees in management. These models should demonstrate collaborative curriculum plan-

ning with other university schools and departments that teach management skills and interdisciplinary management education for nursing, health services administration, and business.

5. Inventories of successful programs and consultation services need to be developed to provide information-sharing, development of theory and guidelines for organizational design, effective management practices for nursing, support service systems, and human resource management.

NURSES AND THE NURSING PROFESSION

Immediate Goals

1. The Nursing profession needs to accelerate efforts to:
   - gain consensus in definition of nursing roles and functions that relate education to practice competencies
   - define fundamental professional goals and policy direction for education and practice
   - ensure competence through admission standards and entry to practice standards
   - develop a commonly understood, unified credentialing system that ensures licensure standards for public safety, provides clear mechanisms for career mobility, and recognizes advanced competencies through certification

2. Nurses should:
   - act collectively through professional associations to create an organized, democratic framework to promote change and improve patient care, and to derive strength to influence health care policies and decisions affecting nursing practice
   - be involved in community, state, and national public interest and policy-making groups for health promotion and other public concerns

3. Nursing organizations and the professional associations need to reach consensus about fundamental professional goals so that:
   - a clear identity of nurses, substantiated in practice, is communicated to the public
   - public policy representatives can relate to the profession's goals in policy initiatives, funding, and regulatory actions
   - career-bound students will be attracted to the nursing profession

NURSES AND UNIONS;
NURSES AND SUPPLEMENTARY STAFFING AGENCIES

Immediate Goals

Health care administrators and nurse administrators need to examine and immediately improve the work setting of nurses. They should:

- assess the adequacy of salaries and benefit programs
- institute flexible scheduling patterns
- develop mechanisms to increase nursing's self-determination in decision-making in the practice setting and to promote its study of performance standards in relation to terms of employment

Research Projects

1. A general and comprehensive study of nurse salaries and working conditions is needed to determine the effects of various mixes of incentives on satisfaction and turnover, such as salary levels and ranges and benefits, flexible scheduling, and weekend and night pay differentials. Sufficient variety of these factors currently exists in health care institutions to conduct an assessment of their effects. A large sample of hospitals is necessary for scientific study.

2. Descriptive and evaluative information is needed on the numbers and types of union organizations representing nurses in collective bargaining activities with health care institutions. Factors to be examined are those associated with the decision to unionize and choice of union; the effects of unionization on salaries; working conditions, and other professional benefits; and conditions under which patient care arrangements, including staffing levels, become a subject for bargaining.

3. Descriptive information is needed on the numbers and types of agencies supplying temporary nursing services to hospitals. Factors to include are features of these arrangements that appeal to nurses, and advantages and disadvantages associated with these arrangements from the perspectives of the health care institution administration, nursing administration, agency nurses, and other nurse employees.

4. Evaluative information is needed to determine the effects of supplemental staffing agencies and alternate forms of employers on the quality of patient care, the implications for nursing staff morale, cost of care, and other critical factors.

THE NURSING PROFESSION
AND NURSING EDUCATION

Immediate Goals

Nurse educators need to examine the nursing education system to:

- develop a clearly defined sequence of nursing education for basic, graduate, and continuing education
- validate competencies of graduates from all types of nursing education programs
- consult with nurses in practice to determine a core curriculum that will establish a consistent and comprehensible base for career advancement in formal and continuing education, and in clinical practice
- coordinate educational programs on a local, state, and regional basis to reduce redundancy in cost and effort, and to ensure availabilty of basic and graduate programs
- preserve existing resources for nursing education and explore ways to combine them into new forms of quality educational programs
- establish flexible programs for registered nurse students and for inactive nurses who may reenter the profession

Accrediting bodies for nursing education need to promote development and implemention of relevant criteria and guidelines that ensure orderly steps in movement of programs from one level of education to another, such as diploma to baccalaureate, and to ensure accessible and flexible programs that meet standards of quality education for registered nurses, nontraditional students and others.

Demonstration Projects

1. Models of cooperative, multiinstitutional programs providing career mobility opportunities from entry level through graduate nursing preparation need to be developed and/or evaluated. Evaluation should measure the effects of these programs on nursing performance, socialization to increasingly complex nursing functions, cost, and other outcomes related to performance and quality patient care.
2. Models of nontraditional nursing education need to be evaluated for their quality and effects in improving educational opportunities for second-career students, registered nurse students, and others; and for their capability to relate education to practice through innovative structures.

NURSING EDUCATION AND NURSING PRACTICE

Immediate Goals

Nurses in education and practice need to examine the appropriate relationship between education and practice by forming mechanisms to develop:

- a clear sequence of education related to nursing practice and one that promotes ease of transition to clinical nursing at basic and graduate levels
- an educational foundation for advanced degrees, continuing education, and career advancement through practice
- opportunities for nurses to pursue full professional roles in clinical practice, education, management, and research in education and practice settings

Demonstration Projects

1. Centers for Nursing could be developed to promote professional interchange and established networks for sharing clinical expertise, nursing practice developments, and other relevant professional concerns by nurses in different types of practice settings and in varying specialties.
2. Models of innovations to ease transition from school to practice should be developed and/or evaluated. These models should relate education to practice, focusing on ways to develop practice competence by establishing realistic clinical performance expectations in education and subsequent development of clinical competence in the practice setting. Externship and internship programs are examples. Attention should be directed to the balance of theory and clinical experience in education and health care institutions' roles in providing educational support and guidance for nurses in practice.

Research Projects

1. The amount of conflict and dissatisfaction exhibited by nurses in the practice setting could be expected to be a function of both expectations and self-conceptions developed in schools and of opportunities provided by practice settings. These predictions could be specified and tested in a sample of nurses drawn from varying educational backgrounds who practice in varying settings.
2. Baccalaureate nursing programs that successfully combine theoretical knowledge with clinical skills could be identified and evaluated to determine the factors that differentiate them from the less successful programs in regard to clinical practice performance.

3. Health care institutions that successfully orient and promote development of clinical knowledge and skill could be identified and evaluated to determine factors necessary to build on basic educational experiences of nurses following graduation.

NURSING AND THE PUBLIC

Immediate Goals

1. Nursing's professional associations need to join in implementing a cooperatively planned national public relations campaign. The support of other health professional groups and organizations should be used in wide dissemination of information that presents a current and realistic image of nursing.
2. Nurses should become active in public policy formulation for health care. They should seek membership on committees and forums for state and national policy and decision-making about health care delivery. They also should become active in community groups that deal with public welfare.
3. The public, legislators, and professional nursing associations need to support national standards for credentialing of nurses.

Demonstration Projects

Models that demonstrate the most effective utilization of nurses with different levels of education in organizational structures appropriate for different types of patients should be developed and/or evaluated to determine cost-effectiveness and quality of care. Information from these models will provide direction in nurse manpower planning.

Research Projects

Cost-effective utilization of nurses could be expected to be a function of matching nursing competencies with patient care needs and the organizational structures in which care takes place. Factors that affect this utilization should be studied, such as management structures, leadership, and educational needs of practicing nurses.

Appendix

REFERENCES

CHAPTER 2: NURSING PRACTICE

Nurses and Physicians; Nurses and Health Care Administrators

1. National Commission on Nursing. *Summary of State Studies and Policy Documents,* Chicago: Hospital Research and Educational Trust, forthcoming.

2. National Association of Nurse Recruiters. 1981 Survey, from Tina Filoromo, speech presented at American Hospital Association Workshop: *Organizing for Nurse Recruiting,* April 1981.

3. Felch, W. C. Physician-Nurse Relationships, *The Hospital Medical Staff,* 6:6-8, July 1976.

4. Kalisch, B. J., and Kalisch, P. A. An Analysis of the Sources of Physician-Nurse Conflict, *Journal of Nursing Administration,* 7:51-7, January 1977.

5. Lewis, Frances Marcus. The Nurse as Lackey: A Sociological Perspective, *Supervisor Nurse,* 7:24-7, April 1976.

6. Lovell, M. C. The Politics of Medical Deception: Challenging the Trajectory of History, *Advanced Nursing Science,* 2:73-86, 1980.

7. Smoyak, S. A. Problems in Interprofessional Relations, *Bulletin of the New York Academy of Medicine,* 53:51-9, January 1977.

8. National Commission on Nursing. *Summary of the Public Hearings.* Chicago: Hospital Research and Educational Trust, 1981.

9. Lee, A. A. Still the Handmaiden, *RN,* 42:21-30, July 1979.

10. Campbell, Gilbert S. Where Are the Nurses of Yesteryear? *American Journal of Surgery,* 133:145, February 1977.

11. Cook, Rosa Lee. Physician-Nurse Collaboration: A Nurse's Perspective, *Aviation, Space, and Environmental Medicine,* 50:1179-81, November 1979.

12. Hoekelman, R. A. Nurse-Physician Relationships, *American Journal of Nursing,* 75:1150-2, July 1975.

13. Richards, R. E. The Games Professionals Play, *Supervisor Nurse,* 9:48-50, June 1978.

14. Sherber, J., and Loder Jr., Robert A. Letting It All Hang Out: How Nurses Rate the Doctors, *RN,* 39:71-4, March 1976.

15. Smoyak, op. cit., Ch. 2, no. 7.

16. Kalisch, B. J., and Kalisch, P. A. Perspectives on Improving Nursing's Public Image, *Nursing and Health Care*, 1:10-18, January 1980.

17. Scher, M., and others. Stereotyping and Role Conflicts Between Medical Students and Psychiatric Nurses, *Health and Community Psychiatry*, 26:219-21, April 1975.

18. National Joint Practice Commission. *Guidelines for Establishing Joint or Collaborative Practice in Hospitals*, Chicago: National Joint Practice Commission, 1981.

19. National Joint Practice Commission. *Statement on the Definition of Joint or Collaborative Practice in Hospitals*, Chicago: National Joint Practice Commission, September 1977.

20. National Joint Practice Commission, op. cit., Ch. 2, no.18.

21. National Commission on Nursing. *Inventory of Innovative Programs and Projects*, Chicago: Hospital Research and Educational Trust, forthcoming.

22. Allen, M., and others. Closing the Communication Gap Between Physicians and Nurses in the Intensive Care Unit Setting, *Heart and Lung*, 9:836-40, September-October 1980.

22. Sherber and Loder, op. cit., Ch. 2, no. 14.

24. Annis, P., and others. Two Professions, Two Perspectives, *Nursing*, 9:33-8, September 1979.

25. Yalof, I. The Multidisciplinary Team: An Effective Approach to Management of the Cardiac Surgery Patient, *Heart and Lung*, 8:699-705, July- August 1979.

26. Taxay, E. P. The Health Care Team, *Journal of the American Medical Association*, 239:1137, December 1978.

27. Bottom, P. A., and others. Administrative Issues in Health Team Development: Report of a Workshop, *Alabama Journal of Medical Sciences*, 14:203-07, February 1977.

28. Gomez, A., and others. Multidisciplinary Team Malfunctioning on a State Hospital Unit: A Case Study, *Hospital and Community Psychiatry*, 31:38-40, January 1980.

29. Frederick, P. E. The Psychiatrist/Psychologist and Team Leader: What About Social Workers and Nurses? *Hospital and Community Psychiatry*, 29:326, May 1978.

30. Vasile, R., and Gutheil, T. The Psychiatrist as Medical Backup: Ambiguity in the Delegation of Clinical Responsibility, *American Journal of Psychiatry*, 136:1292-6, October 1979.

31. Feiger, S., and others. Collegiality in Interdisciplinary Health Teams: Its Measurement and Its Effects, *Social Science and Medicine*, 13A:217-29, 1979.

32. Given, B., and Simmons, S. The Interdisciplinary Health-Care Team: Fact or Fiction? *Nursing Forum*, 16:165-84, 1977.

33. Kane, R. A. The Interprofessional Team as a Small Group, *Social Work and Health Care*, 1:19-32, January 1975.

34. Allen, M. and others. Closing the Communication Gap Between Physicians and Nurses in the Intensive Care Unit Setting, *Heart and Lung*, 9:836-40, 1980.

35. Cunningham, A. Professional Nursing Practice in the Hospital Setting, *Supervisor Nurse*, 11:26, August 1980.

36. Smith, Diane R. What is the Professional Nurse (Really?), *Supervisor Nurse*, 11:34-5, May 1980.

37. Beletz, E. Is Nursing's Public Image Up to Date? *Nursing Outlook,* 22:432-6, July 1974.

38. Chapman, C. M. Image of the Nurse, *International Nursing Review,* 24:166-7, June 1977.

39. Hutchens, C. M. Looking Ahead: Women and Nursing, *Imprint,* 27:74-81, April 27, 1980.

40. Reeder, Sharon J., and Mauksch, Hans. *Nursing: Continuing Change.* In: Freeman, Howard E., Levine, Sol, and Reeder, Leo G., editors, *Handbook of Medical Sociology,* 3rd edition. Englewood Cliffs, NJ: Prentice-Hall, Inc., 1979.

41. Smith, op. cit., Ch. 2, no. 36.

42. Donovan, L. What Nurses Want (And What They're Getting), *RN,* 43:22-30, April 1980.

43. Price, J. L., and Mueller, C. W. *Professional Turnover: The Case of Nurses.* NY: SP Medical and Scientific Books, 1981.

44. Brief, Arthur P. Turnover Among Hospital Numbers: A Suggested Model. *Journal of Nursing Administration,* 6:55-7, October 1976.

45. Cronin-Stubbs, D. Job Satisfaction and Dissatisfaction Among New Graduate Staff Nurses, *The Journal of Nursing Administration,* 7:44-9, December 1977.

46. Araujo, Marianne. Creative Nursing Administration Sets Climate for Retention, *Hospitals,* 54:72-6, May 1, 1980.

Nurses and Health Care Institutions

47. National Commission on Nursing, op. cit., Ch. 2, no.1.

48. Cronin-Stubbs, op. cit., Ch. 2, no. 45.

49. Fly, K. Job Satisfaction Factors for Nurses in a Pediatric Hospital Research study report, Corpus Christi (TX) State University, December 16, 1980.

50. Long, A., and Mercer, G. The Turnover of Labour in Nursing, *Health Services Manpower Review,* 3:6-10, December 1977.

51. Strilaeff, F. Supervision and Turnover of General Staff Nurses, *Dimensions in Health Services,* 53:36-9, November 1976.

52. Weisman, C. S., and others. *Job Satisfaction and Turnover Among Hospital Nurses. Final Report.* School of Hygiene and Public Health. The Johns Hopkins University, November 1979.

53. American Society for Nursing Service Administrators. Profile of the Nursing Service Administrator Revisited: A Preliminary Report Based on an Analysis of Gross Data from the *1977 Survey of Nursing Service Administrators in Hospitals,* March 1980.

54. Sample, S. A. Development of Organizational Bylaws, An Approach to Accountability, *Nursing Clinics of North America,* 13:91-102, March 1978.

55. Spitzer, Roxanne. The Nurse and the Corporate World, *Supervisor Nurse,* 12:21-4, April 1981.

56. Christman, L. The Autonomous Nursing Staff in the Hospital, *Nursing Administration Quarterly,* 1:37-44, Fall 1976.

57. Kimbro, C. D., and Gifford, A. J. The Nursing Staff Organization: A Needed Development, *Nursing Outlook,* 28:610-16, October 1980.

58. Symons, B. Rose Nursing Congress Aids Voice in Role Determination, *Denver Post,* May 31, 1981.

59. Christman, op. cit., Ch. 2, no. 56.

60. Cleland, V. S. Shared Governance in a Professional Model of Collective Bargaining, *Journal of Nursing Administration,* 8:39-43, May 1978.

61. Kenwood, N. J., and VanCura, B. On the Scene: Organizational Structures of Nursing Services at Northwestern Memorial Hospital, *Nursing Administration Quarterly,* 3:12-18, Spring 1979.

62. Martel, G., and others. On the Scene: Organizational Structures of Nursing Services at Northwestern Memorial Hospital, *Nursing Administration Quarterly,* 3:11-23, Winter 1979.

63. Davis, Anne J. Nursing's Influence on Health Policy for the Eighties. In: American Academy of Nursing, Scientific Session, *Nursing's Influence on Health Policy for the Eighties.* American Nurses' Association, Kansas City, MO: 1979.

64. Ehrenreich, Barbara, and Ehrenreich, John H. Hospital Workers: Class Conflicts in the Making, *International Journal of Health Services,* 5:43-51, January 1975.

65. Kinney, Marguerite. Professional-Bureaucratic Conflicts, *Heart and Lung,* 8:1025-6, November-December 1979.

66. Martin, Jean-Claude. Hospital Problems Need Interprofessional Approach, *Dimensions in Health Service,* 56:8, August 1979.

67. Spencer, Conby E. Nurses Need Liberation—But From Whom? *RN,* 42:63-4, July 1979.

68. Tebbitt, B. V. Preparing the Interviewer, *Supervisor Nurse,* 8:45-8, April 1977.

69. National Commission on Nursing, op. cit., Ch. 2, no. 8.

70. Carey, R. G. Evaluation of a Primary Nursing Unit, *American Journal of Nursing,* 79:1253-5, July 1979.

71. Corpuz, T. Primary Nursing Meets Needs, Expectations of Patient and Staff, *Hospitals,* 51:95-100, June 1, 1977.

72. Daeffler, R. J. Patients' Perception of Care Under Team and Primary Nursing, *Journal of Nursing Administration,* 5:20-6, March-April 1975.

73. Donahue, Mary, and others. Dreams and Realities, a Nurse, Physician and Administrator View Primary Nursing, *Nursing Clinics of North America,* 12:247-55, June 1977.

74. Durham, R. C. A Plan for Researching the Effects of Primary Nursing Care. (From: The Realities of Primary Nursing Care: Risk, Roles, Reasearch; New York: NLN, 1978) pp.45-50. Paper presented at Southern Regional Assembly of Constituent Leagues of the National League for Nursing in Atlanta, Georgia, November 1977.

75. Werner, J., editor. The Evanston Story: Primary Nursing Comes Alive, *Nursing Administration Quarterly,* 1:9-50, Winter 1977.

76. Christman, Luther. Current Roles of Nursing in Health Care, *Southern Medical Journal,* 70:264-5, March 1977.

77. Nursing Administrative Action on the Management Team, *Journal of Nursing Administration,* 8:37-8, December 1978.

78. Dickerson, T. Introduction. (From: The Realities of Primary Nursing Care: Risk, Roles, Research; New York: NLN, 1978). pp.1-4. Paper presented at Southern Regional Assembly of Constituent Leagues of National League for Nursing in Atlanta, GA, November 1977.

79. Russell, R. C. Rationale for Primary Nursing Care. (From: Primary Nursing: One Nurse, One Client, Planning Care Together; New York: NLN, 1977) pp. 11-17. Paper presented at Southern Regional Assembly of Constituent Leagues of the National League for Nursing in Atlanta, GA, December 1976-January 1977.

80. Sheard, Timothy. The Structure of Conflict in Nurse-Physician Relations, *Supervisor Nurse,* 11:14-18, August 1980.

81. Williams, F. G., and Stewart, M. T. Pilot Unit Shifts to Primary Nursing, *Hospitals,* 54:112-15, January 16, 1980.

82. Alexander, C. S., and others. Evaluating Primary Nursing in Hospitals: Examination of Effects on Nursing Staff, *Medical Care,* 19:80-9, January 1981.

83. Anderson, M., and Denyes, M. A Ladder for Clinical Advancement in Nursing Practice: Implementation, *Journal of Nursing Administration,* 5:16-22, February 1975.

84. Bernal, H. Levels of Practice in a Community Health Agency, *Nursing Outlook,* 26:364-9, June 1978.

85. Bracken, R. L., and Christman, L. An Incentive Program Designed to Develop and Reward Clinical Competence, *Journal of Nursing Administration,* 8:8-18, October 1978.

86. Colavecchio, R., and others. A Clinical Ladder for Nursing Practice, *Journal of Nursing Administration,* 4:54-8, September-October 1974.

87. Meintel, P., and Rhodes, D. Clinical Career Ladder Rewards RNs, *Hospital Progress,* 58:36-47, August 1977.

88. Bernal, op. cit., Ch. 2, no. 84.

89. Colavecchio, and others, op. cit., Ch. 2, no. 86.

Nurses and the Nursing Profession

90. Greenwood, E. The Elements of Professionalization. In: Vollmer, H. M., and Mills, D. L., editors. *Professionalization.* Englewood Cliffs, NJ: Prentice-Hall, Inc., 1965, pp. 9-20.

91. Caplow, T. The Sequence of Professionalization. In: Vollmer, H. M., and Mills, D. L., editors. *Professionalization.* Englewood Cliffs, NJ: Prentice-Hall, Inc., 1965, pp. 19-21.

92. Wilensky, H. L. The Professionalization of Everyone? *American Journal of Sociology,* 70:137-58, September 1964.

93. Hughes, E. C. The Social Contest of Professionalization. In: Vollmer, H. M., and Mills, D. L., editors. *Professionalization.* Englewood Cliffs, NJ: Prentice-Hall Inc., 1966, pp. 64-70.

94. Schulman, S. Mother Surrogate—After a Decade. In: Gortly Jaco, E., editor. *Patients, Physicians and Illness.* 3rd edition. New York: The Free Press, 1979.

95. Johnston, T. The Sexist in Nursing: Who is She? *Nursing Forum,* 18:204-05, 1979.

96. Keller, M. C. The Effect of Sexual Stereotyping on the Development of Nursing Theory, *American Journal of Nursing,* 79:1585-6, September 1979.

97. Kelley, L. K., and Baker, J. M. Women in Nursing and Academic Tenure, *Journal of Nursing Education,* 19:41-8, March-April 1980.

98. Brown, S. P. Some Concerns on Certification, *Association of Operating Room Nurses Journal,* 31:51-2, January 1980.

99. DeTornay, T. The Task Ahead—Acceptance and Implementation. *AORN Journal,* 31:53, January 1980.

100. Gunn, I. P. Certification for Specialty Practice, *AORN Journal,* 31:48-51, January 1980.

101. *The Study of Credentialing in Nursing: A New Approach,* vol. 1. The Report of the Committee, Kansas City, MO: American Nurses' Association, Publication Code G-1365M, March 1979.

102. Seldon, W. K. The Study Can Bring Together Nursing Leadership, *AORN Journal*, 31:47-8, January 1980.

103. National Commission on Nursing, op. cit., Ch. 2, no. 1.

104. Ibid.

105. Council on Higher Education. *Kentucky Report presented to National Commission on Nursing.* Atlanta, GA: February 27, 1981.

106. McConnell, W. R. *High School Graduates: Projection for the Fifty States.* Boulder, CO: Western Interstate Commission on Higher Education, 1979.

107. U.S. Department of Health, Education, and Welfare. *Special Report on Aging:* 1979 DHEW Pub. No. CNIH 79-1907, 1979.

Nurses and Unions; Nurses and Supplementary Staffing Agencies

108. Brief, op. cit., Ch. 2, no. 44.

109. Cronin-Stubbs, op. cit., Ch. 2, no. 45.

110. Howell, D. L., and Steward, G. T. Labor Turnover in Hospitals, *Personnel Journal*, 54:624-7, December 1975.

111. Long and Mercer, op. cit., Ch. 2, no. 50.

112. Ordell, H., and Woods, G. L. Coping with the Nursing Shortage, *Health Services Manager,* 13:4, April 1980.

113. National Commission on Nursing, op. cit., Ch. 2, no. 1.

114. White, C. H. Nursing Shortage, Turnover and Some Proposed Solutions, *Hospital Forum,* 22:10-13, June 1979.

115. Mulcahy, R. W., and Radar, D. W. Trends in Hospital Labor Relations, *Topics in Health Care Financing,* 6:57-73, Spring 1980.

116. Tanner, L. D., and others. Collective Bargaining in the Health Care Industry, *Monthly Labor Review,* pp. 49-53, February 1980.

117. Mulcahy and Radar, op, cit., Ch. 2, no. 115.

118. Sheahan, R. E. Can Southern Hospitals Fight the Unions? *Southern Hospitals,* 48:12-16, January-February 1980.

119. Hopkins, J. H., and Binderup, R. D. Union Elections Are Seldom Won or Lost During the Campaign, *The Personnel Administrator,* pp. 57-61, March 1980.

120. Hopping, B. Professionalism and Unionism: Conflicting Ideologies, *Nursing Forum,* 15:372-83, 1976.

121. Hill, C. A. The Void in Collective Bargaining: Professional Employees, *The Personnel Administrator,* August 1979.

122. DeMarko, K., and others. A Pilot Study of the Initial Bargaining Demands by Newly-Organized Employees of Health Care Institutions, *Labor Law Journal,* pp. 275-91, May 1978.

123. Godfrey, M. A. Nurses' Salaries Today, *Nursing '77,* 7:81-97, June 1977.

124. Helin, E. B. Negotiating a Professional Nurses' Contract, *Hospital Topics,* 56:24-8, March -April 1978.

125. Lucas, A. L. What's Nursing Worth? *RN,* 43:31-183, January 1980.

126. Telesco, M. Let's Say Yes to Unions, *RN,* 41:29-34, November 1978.

127. Wynne, D. A Union Contract Was the Only Language Our Hospital Would Understand, *RN,* 41:66-8, May 1978.

128. Godfrey, op. cit., Ch. 2, no. 123.

129. Lucas, op. cit., Ch. 2, no. 125.

130. Moore, T. F. Union Decertification: Bucking the Trend, *Hospital Topics,* 55:14-15, May-June 1977.

131. Natonski, J. Why a Union Contract Didn't Work at Our Hospital, *RN*, 41:69-71, May 1978.
132. Reece, A. Union Decertification and the Salaried Approach: A Workable Alternative, *Journal of Nursing Administration*, 7:20-4, July-August 1977.
133. Jett, M. Use of Temporary Nursing Personnel as Cost-Control Measure, *Hospital Topics*, 55:48-50, July-August 1977.
134. Ibid.
135. Thompson, D. Supplemental Staffing: Can It Be Cost-Effective? *Hospitals*, 55:74-7, March 16, 1981.

CHAPTER 3: NURSING EDUCATION

The Nursing Profession and Nursing Education

1. Johnson, W. L. Supply and Demand for Registered Nurses: Some Observations on the Current Picture and Prospects to 1985, *Nursing and Health Care*, August 1980.
2. Ibid.
3. Vaughn, J. C. Educational Preparation for Nursing—1979, *Nursing and Health Care*, 1:6, September 1980.
4. Roth, A., and others. 1977 national sample survey of registered nurses: a report on the nurse population and factors affecting their supply. Kansas City: American Nurses' Association, 1979.
5. National Commission on Nursing, op. cit., Ch. 2, no. 1.
6. Ibid.
7. Cobin, J. T. RN Educational Mobility is Goal of Consortium, *Hospitals*, 54:87-91, November 1, 1980.
8. National Commission on Nursing, op. cit., Ch. 2, no. 1.
9. Richard Steele Consultants, Inc. *The Diploma School of Nursing in the 1980's*. A report to the Association of Diploma Schools of Nursing in Connecticut, March 1979.
10. Roth, op. cit., Ch. 3, no. 4.
11. National League for Nursing, Division of Research. *NLN Nursing Data Book*. New York: NLN, Pub. No. 19-1751, 1978.
12. *Inactive Nurse Study*, Virginia State Department of Health, August 1980.
13. Indiana Commission for Higher Education. *Recommendations for Nursing Education*, January 1981.
14. Cobin, op. cit, Ch. 2, no. 7.
15. Open Forums sponsored by National Commission on Nursing and the Center for Small or Rural Hospitals, American Hospital Association, April-May 1981.
16. Mauksch, I. G. Faculty Practice: A Professional Imperative, *Nurse Educator*, 5:21-4, May-June 1980.
17. Felton, G. *Is Academic Nursing Preparing Practitioners to Meet Present and Future Societal Needs?* Publication Series 81(1), American Association of Colleges of Nursing, October 1980.
18. Brown, B., and others. A Costing Methodology for Schools of Nursing, *Nursing Outlook*, 27:584-9, September 1979.
19. Derby, V. L. Financing Nursing Education, *Nurse Educator*, 5:21-5, March-April 1980.

20. Prescott, P., and Sorensen, J. E. Cost-Effective Analysis: An Approach to Evaluating Nursing Programs, *NAQ*, 3:17-40, Fall 1978.

21. Simonds, S. K. Quality, Accountability, and Professional Responsibility: New Tasks for Inservice Education Directors, *The Journal of Continuing Education in Nursing*, 6:5-11, July-August 1975.

22. Gilliss, C. L. Teaching Group Skills to Nurse Managers, *The Journal of Continuing Education in Nursing*, 10:19-30, May-June 1979.

23. Kase, S., and Swenson, B. *Costs of Hospital-Sponsored Orientation and Inservice Education for Registered Nurses.* DHEW Pub. No. HRA 77-25, November 1976.

24. Hicks, G., and White, C. The Cost of Orienting and Retaining Nurses, *CHA Insight*, 5:1-4, California Hospital Association, June 4, 1981.

25. Calkin, J. D. Let's Rethink Staff Development Programs. *The Journal of Nursing Administration*, 9:16-19, June 1979.

26. Nodell, C. Why Inservice Education? *Long Term Care and Health Services Administration Quarterly*, 1:33-44, March 1977.

27. Simonds, op. cit., Ch. 3, no. 21.

28. Tobin, H. Quality Staff Development: A Must for Change and Survival, *JONA*, 6:39-42, May 1976.

29. Croll, K. Philosophical Considerations for Inservice Education, *The Journal of Continuing Education in Nursing*, 8:24-6, September-October 1977.

30. Poole, D. Roles and Function of Staff Development Directors, *The Journal of Continuing Education in Nursing*, 8:31-41, May-June 1977.

31. Open Forums, op. cit., Ch. 3, no.15.

32. del Bueno, D. J. Organizing and Staffing the Inservice Department, *JONA*, 6:12-13, December 1976.

33. King, P. J. The Hospitalwide Education Department, *JONA*, 8:4, April 1978.

34. Hicks, B. C., and others. A Need-Oriented Approach to Staff Development, *JONA*, 7:46-7, September 1977.

35. Kent, L., and others. On the Scene, Staff Development at University Hospital, University of Washington, *Nursing Administration Quarterly*, 4:11-52, Fall 1979.

36. White, M. B., and Coburn, D. The Trials, Tribulations, and Triumphs of Curriculum Change, *Nursing Outlook*, 25:644-9, October 1977.

37. Frederickson, K. C., and Mayer, G. H. G. Problem-solving Skills: What Effect has Education? *American Journal of Nursing*, 77:1167-9, July 1977.

38. Gray, J. E., and others. Do Graduates of Technical and Professional Nursing Programs Differ in Practice? *Nursing Research*, 26:368-73, September-October 1977.

39. Bollough, B., and Sparks, C. Baccalaureate vs. Associate Degree Nurses: The Care—Cure Dichotomy, *Nursing Outlook*, 23:688-92, November 1975.

40. Petti, E. R. A Study of the Relationships Between the Three Levels of Nursing Education and Nurse Competency as Rated by Patient and Head Nurse. Dissertation Abstracts International, Boston University, 1975.

41. Nelson, L. F. Competence of Nursing Graduates in Technical, Communicative and Administrative Skills, *Nursing Research*, 27:121-5, March-April 1978.

42. Davis, C. *Relation of University Preparation to Nursing Practice*, NLN Pub. no. 15-1583, 1975.

43. Behm, R. J., and Warnock, F. N. State Board Examinations and Associate Degree Program Effectiveness, *Nursing Research*, 27:54-6, January-February 1978.

44. Knopf, L. *RNs One and Five Years After Graduation.* New York: NLN, 1975.

45. Copeland, W. L., and Miller, B. E. Development of a Modular Curriculum for Nursing Service Orientation, *The Journal of Continuing Education in Nursing,* 7:10-15, July-August 1976.

46. Martin, P. D. The Graduate Nurse Transition Program, *Supervisor Nurse,* 7:18-22, December 1976.

47. Guida, F. K. Treating the Orientation Overload System, *Supervisor Nurse,* 8:28-31, October 1977.

48. Montag, M. Looking Back: Associate Degree Education in Perspective, *Nursing Outlook,* 28:248-50, April 1980.

49. Christman, L., Current Roles of Nursing in Health Care, *Southern Medical Journal,* 70:264-5, March 1977.

50. Benner, P., and others. *From Novice to Expert: A Community View of Preparing for and Rewarding Excellence in Clinical Practice,* University of San Francisco, January 16, 1981.

51. National Commission on Nursing, op. cit., Ch. 2, no. 21.

52. Limon, S., and others. A Clinical Preceptorship to Prepare Reality-Based ADN Graduates, *Nursing and Health Care,* 2:267-9, May 1981.

53. Dexter, P. A., and Laidig, J. Breaking the Educational Service Barrier, *Nursing Outlook,* 28:179-82, March 1980.

54. Pardue, S. F. Blocked and Integrated Content Baccalaureate Nursing Programs, *Nursing Research,* 28:305-11, September-October 1979.

55. Veith, S. Rethinking the Integrated Curriculum, *Nursing Outlook,* 26:187-90, March 1978.

56 Feeley, E., and Tarr, J. Alternative Leadership Experiences for Senior Students in an Acute Care Setting, *Journal of Nursing Education,* 18:25-8, February 1979.

57. Coco, C. D. A Report on Nurse Internship Programs, *Supervisor Nurse,* 7:12-16, December 1976.

58. Holloran, S. D., and others. Bicultural Training for New Graduates, *Nurse Educator,* 5:8-14, January-February 1980.

59. Porter, S. F. Interaction Modeling: An Educational Strategy for New Graduate Leadership Development, *JONA,* 8:20-4, April 1978.

60. Hohman, J. Nurse Mentor System Cuts Costs, Boosts Quality of Care, *Hospitals,* 53:93-101, January 1, 1979.

61. del Bueno, D. J., and Kelly, K. J. How Cost-Effective is Your Staff Development Program? *JONA,* 10:31-6, April 1980.

62. Dinsmore, V. K., and others. Credit for Faculty Practice Model: A Proposal, *Nursing and Health Care,* 2:17-21, January 1981.

63. Lerner, W. M., and Hejna, W. F. Faculty/Staff Contracts: An Alternative for Academic Medical Centers, *Health Care Management Review,* pp. 27-32, Spring 1979.

64. Orden, S. R., and others. Service, Teaching, and Research in a University Ambulatory Care Facility, *Journal of Ambulatory Care Management,* May 1980.

65. National Commission on Nursing, op. cit., Ch. 2, no. 21.

66. Bloch, D. Criteria, Standards, Norms, *JONA,* 7:20-30, September 1977.

67. Young, J., and others. *A Comparative Study of Team and Primary Nursing Care on Two Surgical Inpatient Units.* Baltimore: Johns Hopkins University, 1980.

79

68. Ramphal, M. Rethinking Diploma School and Collegiate Education, *Nursing Outlook*, 26:768-71, December 1978.

69. Nyberg, J., and Simler, M. Developing a Framework for an Integrated Department, *JONA*, 9:9-15, November 1979.

70. Open Forums, op. cit., Ch. 3, no. 15.

71. Smith, R. B. Innovative Programs Keep Them Down on the Farm, *Hospitals*, 16:131-4, March 16, 1979.

72. Moscovice, I. The Influence of Training Level and Practice Setting on Patterns of Primary Care Provided by Nursing Personnel, *Journal of Community Health*, 4:4-14, Fall 1978.

73. del Bueno, D. J., and Kelly, K. J. How Cost-Effective is Your Staff Development Program? *JONA*, 10:31-36, April 1980.